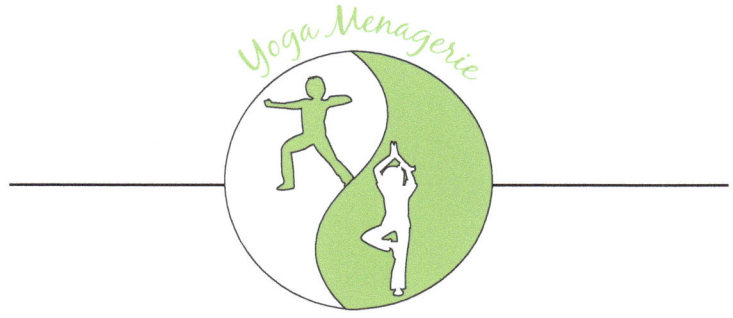

For My Children

Drake and Zoe;

May You Always Follow Your Flow

Yoga Menagerie's
ADVENTURES IN
KIDS YOGA
Book One

BY: VICTORIA FISHMAN
ILLUSTRATED BY: MORGAN KELLER

Yoga Menagerie's Adventures in Kids Yoga is a fun, innovative program that is designed to equip children with the skills they need to reach thier full potential through yoga. They are based on a vinyasa or "flow" yoga, which uses fluid movements and breathing techniques to keep kids engaged in balance between movement and stillness. They are suitable for all ages, levels and abilities and can increase in difficulty with pose variation when necessary. *Yoga Menagerie's Adventures in Kids Yoga explores over 100 Yoga Poses!*

Performing Yoga Menagerie's Adventures in Kids Yoga helps to develop flexibility, strength, balance, coordination, rhythm, stamina, physical awareness and many other gross motor development skills. These adventures bring awareness of the mind-body connection and promote self-discipline and inner strength. They also help to discover and improve relaxation and self-soothing skills; such as coping with stress and other difficult emotions.

Yoga Menagerie's Adventures in Kids Yoga increases concentration, focus and memory development while building self-esteem and encouraging creative imagination and self-expression and promote a positive attitude towards exercise and fitness. Yoga Menagerie's Adventures in Kids Yoga allows everyone to follow their own flow. Use these adventures to learn to flow together!

This book contains an amazing alphabetized picture glossary to help you learn and explain the poses. It also includes a special section for Yoga Journaling so everyone can chart their progress and record their experiences.

This book also contains a chapter designed to enhance breathing practices. These sequences are inspired by pranayama exercises and designed to allow exploration into the different breathing techniques in a kid and family-friendly way.

ALL YOU HAVE TO DO IS SAY THE WORDS AND DO THE YOGA POSES;
JUST FOLLOW ALONG WITH THE FLOW AND HAVE FUN!

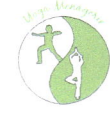

The Adventure Guide

ADVENTURES IN KIDS YOGA (BOOK ONE)

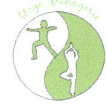

ADVENTURES IN KIDS YOGA

Chapter One

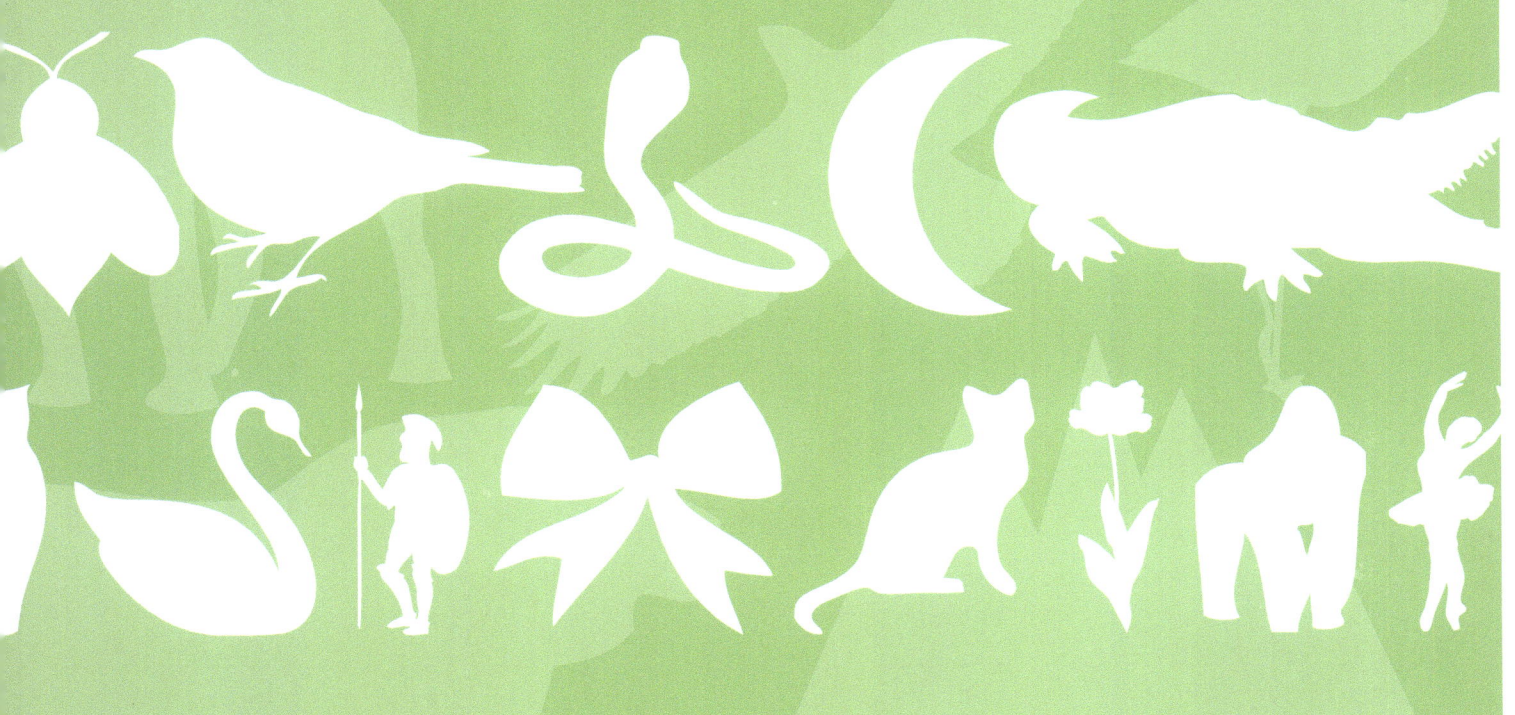

Hello Sun!

FOR THE SUN SALUTATIONS SEQUENCE

Hello Sun! How do you do? We want to say Good Day to you!	*Mountain/Palm Press* *Palm Press –up*
We reach up high to do this pose; Then bend down low and touch our toes.	*Reach up* *Bend to touch toes*
Up a bit to touch our knees; Down to plank now if you please.	*Touch knees-flat back* *Plank*
Spread your feet to be a croc; Then a snake hiding by a rock.	*Crocodile* *Cobra*
Now pretend to be a pup; Then warriors with their swords up.	*Down Dog* *Warrior*
Last, stand up tall and true; Our greeting to the sun is thru.	*Mountain/Palm Press* *Mountain*

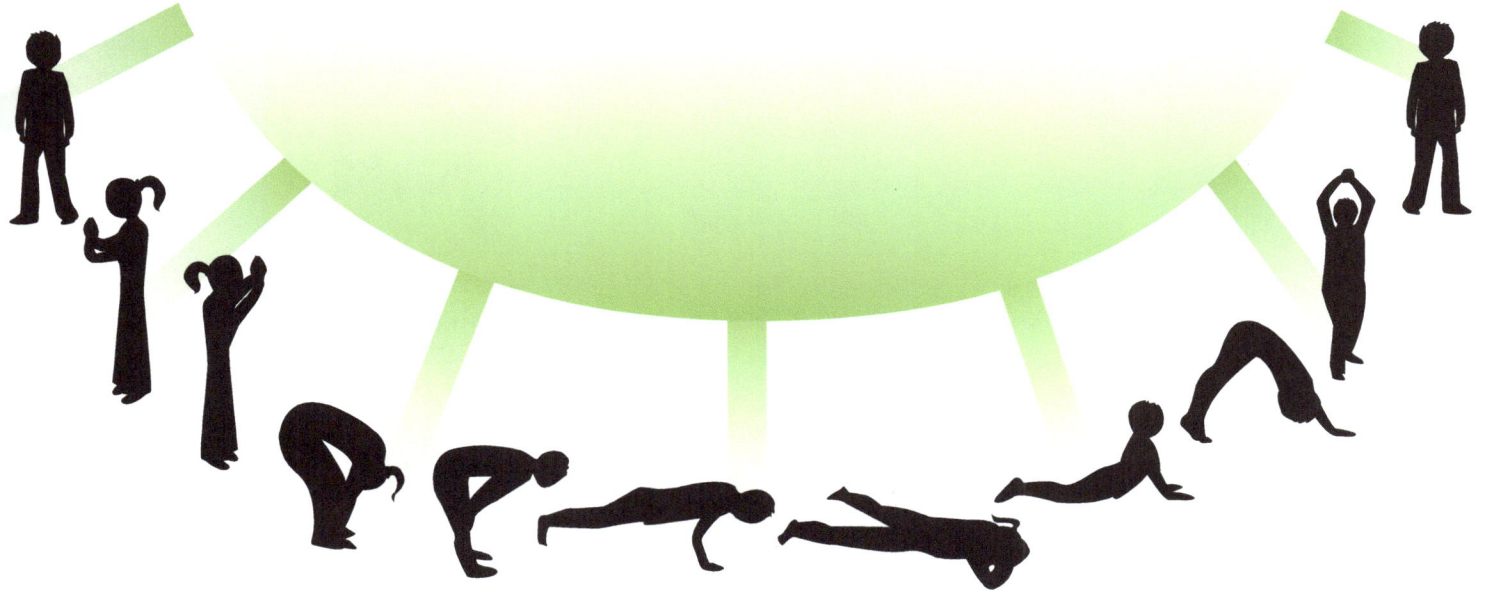

Hello Moon!
FOR THE MOON SALUTATION

It's time to say Hello to the Moon;   *Palm Press- up*
You know the night is coming soon.   *Crescent Moon – Right*
The moon shines down upon the ground;   *Open Hero - Right*
As the stars sparkle all around.   *Star*
We reach over and touch one toe;   *Triangle*
Then the other - down we go.   *Head to knee*
Bend one knee and then face front;   *Lunge /Forward Lunge*
Come to the middle - then mix it up.   *Squat /Forward Lunge*
Turn and face the other way;   *Lunge to the right*
Lift up and straighten, but only halfway.   *Head to Knee - right*
Now twist up - reach for the sky;   *Triangle*
Then be a star floating by.   *Star*
The moon shines down on the Earth so bright; *Open Hero - Left*
Sharing with us its beautiful light.   *Crescent Moon –Left*
Saying Hello to the Moon was fun;   *Palm Press*
Now we've finished where we begun.   *Mountain*

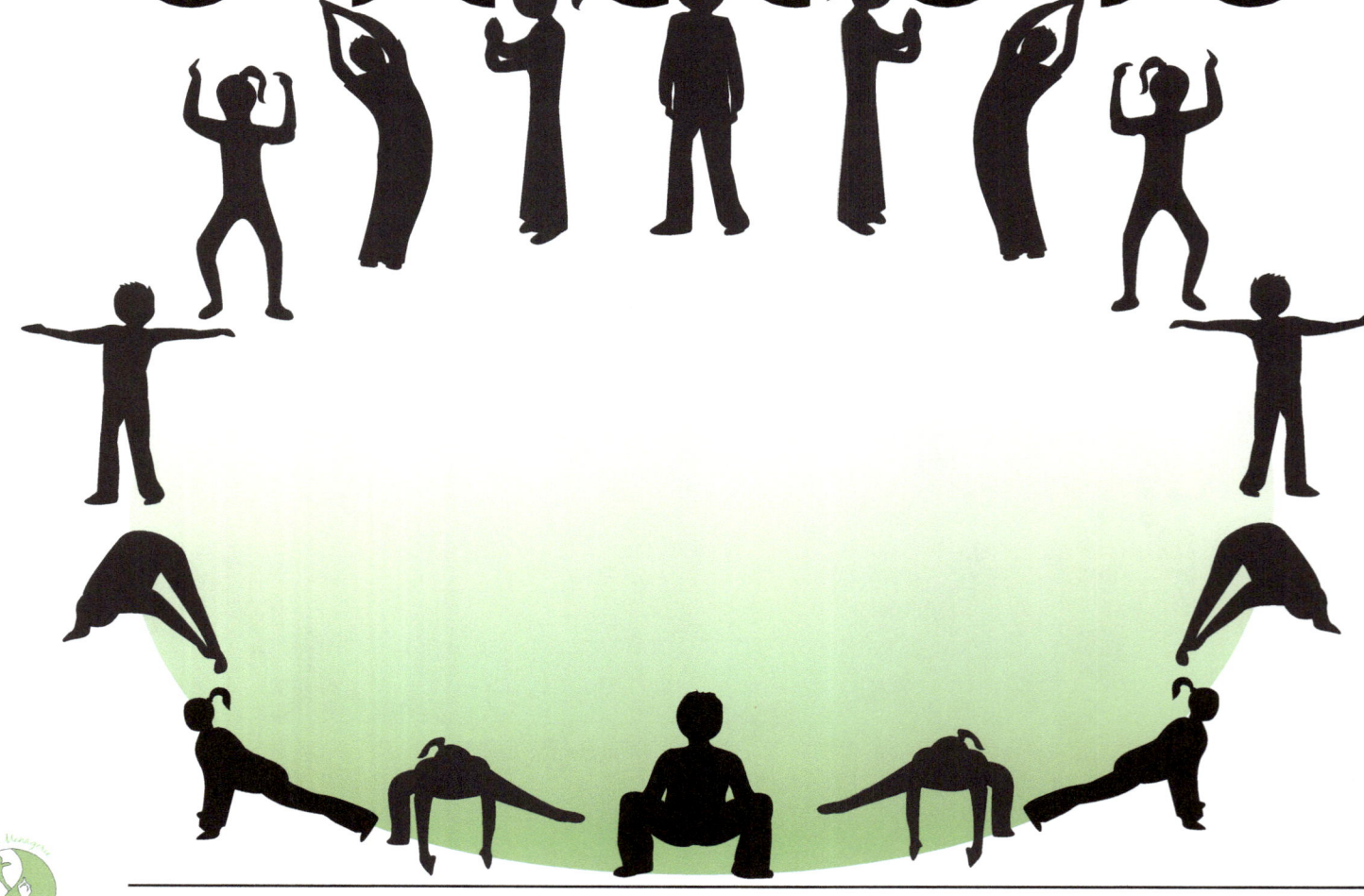

Yoga Numbers

I can make the numbers one thru ten,	*1-10*
Using yoga to stretch and bend.	*Crescent moon*
The number one is nice and tall;	*Mountain*
But two is tricky...Be careful not to fall.	*Cactus*
Three is easy as can be;	*Chair*
And number four looks like a tree.	*Tree*
To be a five we bend our knees,	*Bend knees*
And lift our arms in front with ease.	*Lift arms in front*
We stand up tall to be a six,	*Dancer*
Stretch like a dancer ... just like this.	
The number seven is up next,	*Side stretch*
To do this one... we bend and flex	
The number eight is very round;	*Round arms/Bent legs*
And number nine leans toward the ground.	*Mt – side stretch*
Last we do the number ten,	*Mountain*
Stand up tall, then roll around again.	*Armadillo*
Those are the numbers one thru ten,	*1-10*
Yoga's so much fun, let's do it again!	*Star*

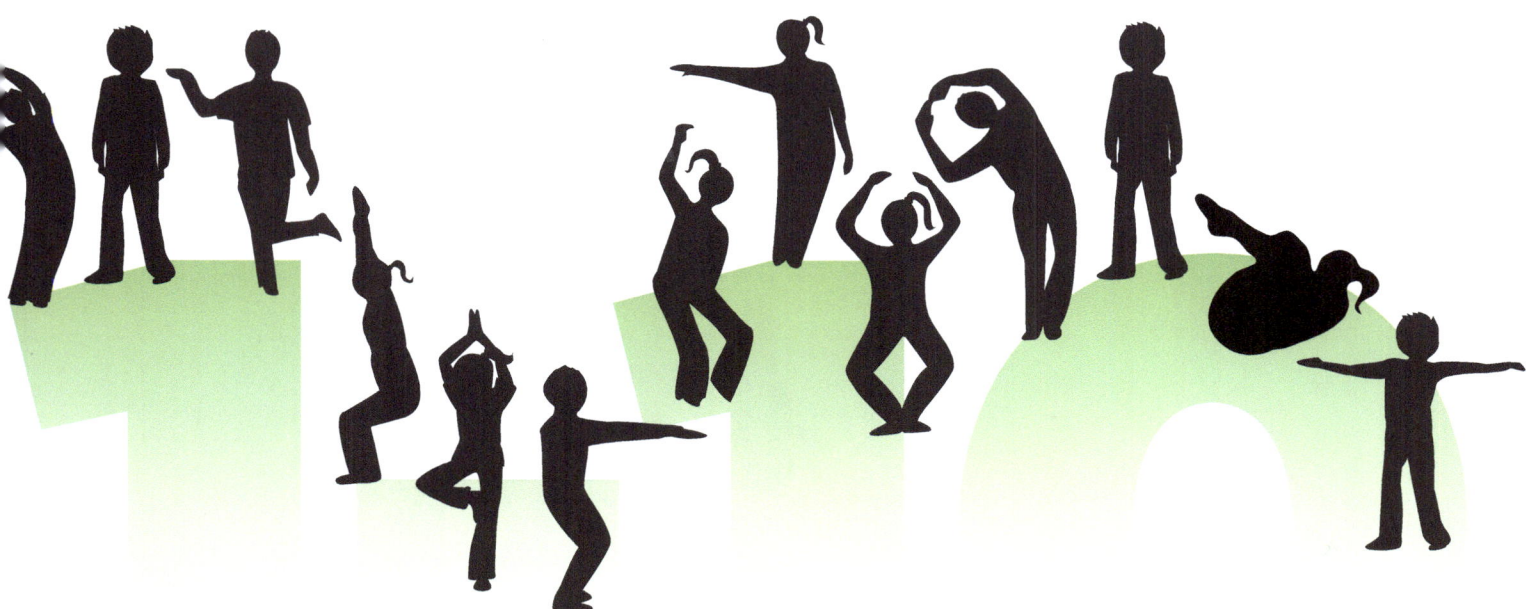

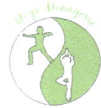

The Yoga Birds
HELP ME TO TAKE FLIGHT

The Yoga Birds help me to take flight,	*Bird - Right*
And follow the flow until everything's right.	*Bird - Left*
The Flamingo balances on just one leg,	*Flamingo*
He switches them fast and does it again.	*Reverse*
The Eagle soars up very high;	*Eagle*
Stretching his wings up to the sky.	*Arms out to side*
The Peacock seems so very small,	*Peacock - lunge*
Until he lifts his feathers tall.	*Lift arms*
The big-eyed Owl twists around,	*Owl*
Looking for mice down on the ground.	*Reverse*
The Pigeon reaches one leg back,	*Pigeon*
And puffs his chest out - just like that.	*Lift Back up*
The Swan is graceful, sleek and white,	*Swan*
She is such a beautiful sight.	
The Yoga Birds help me to take flight,	*Bird*
And follow the flow until everything's right.	

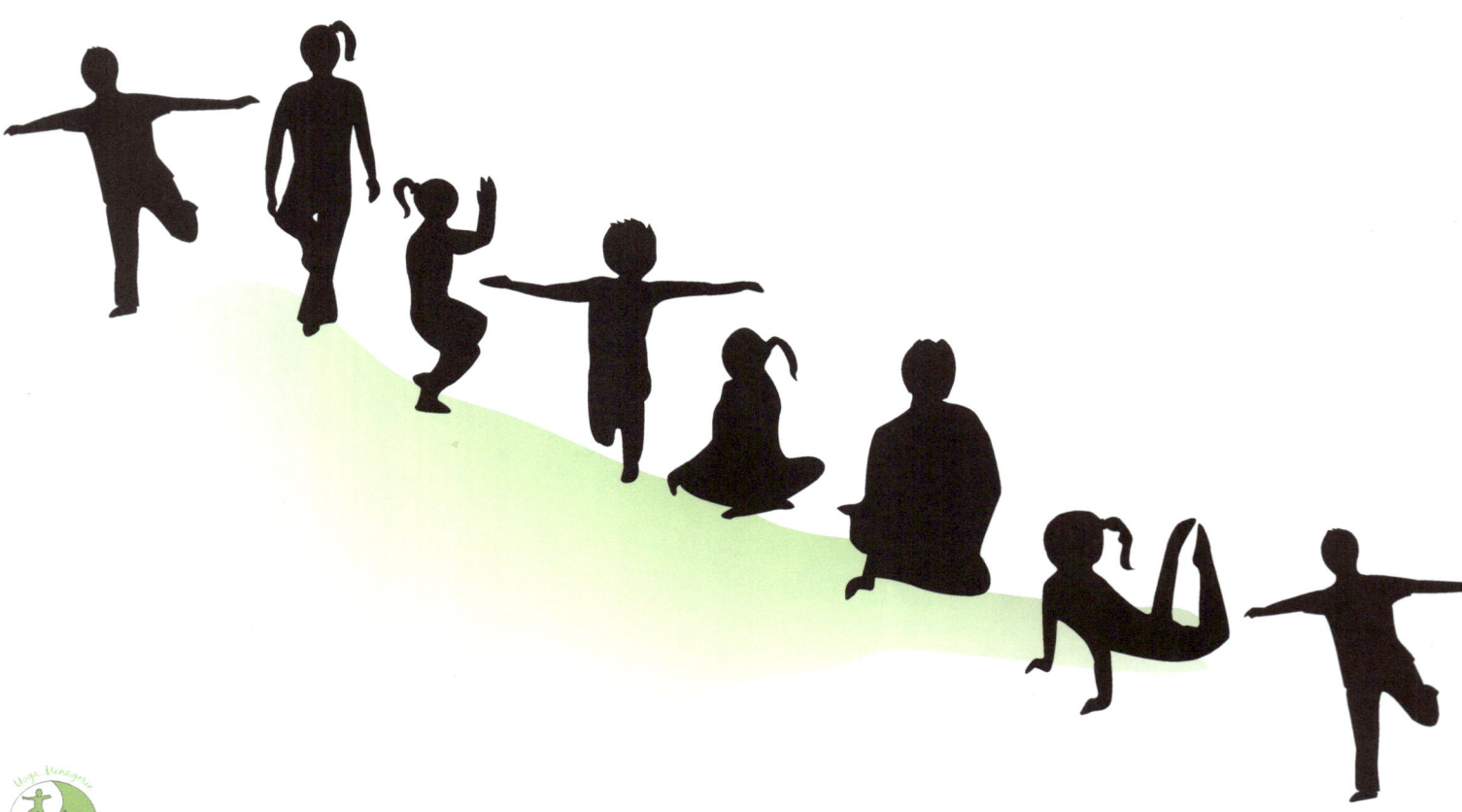

ADVENTURES IN KIDS YOGA

Chapter Two

Focus with Nature

When I feel a little nervous;	*Open Hero*
I use the Earth to help me focus.	
I think of lightening from up so high;	*Lightening – Chair*
And of the rains falling from the sky.	*Rain – Waterfall*
I think of tiny little seeds,	*Seed – Squat*
And how they grow into big trees.	*Tree*
I think of the moon and how it shines so bright;	*Crescent Moon – Right*
It lights up the night with all of its might.	*Crescent Moon – Left*
I think of the stars twinkling above;	*Star*
Filling the sky with all of their love.	
I think of mountains on a great plateau;	*Mountain*
And of an erupting volcano.	*Volcano*
But my favorite place to sit and stop;	*Rock*
Is on my special thinking rock!	

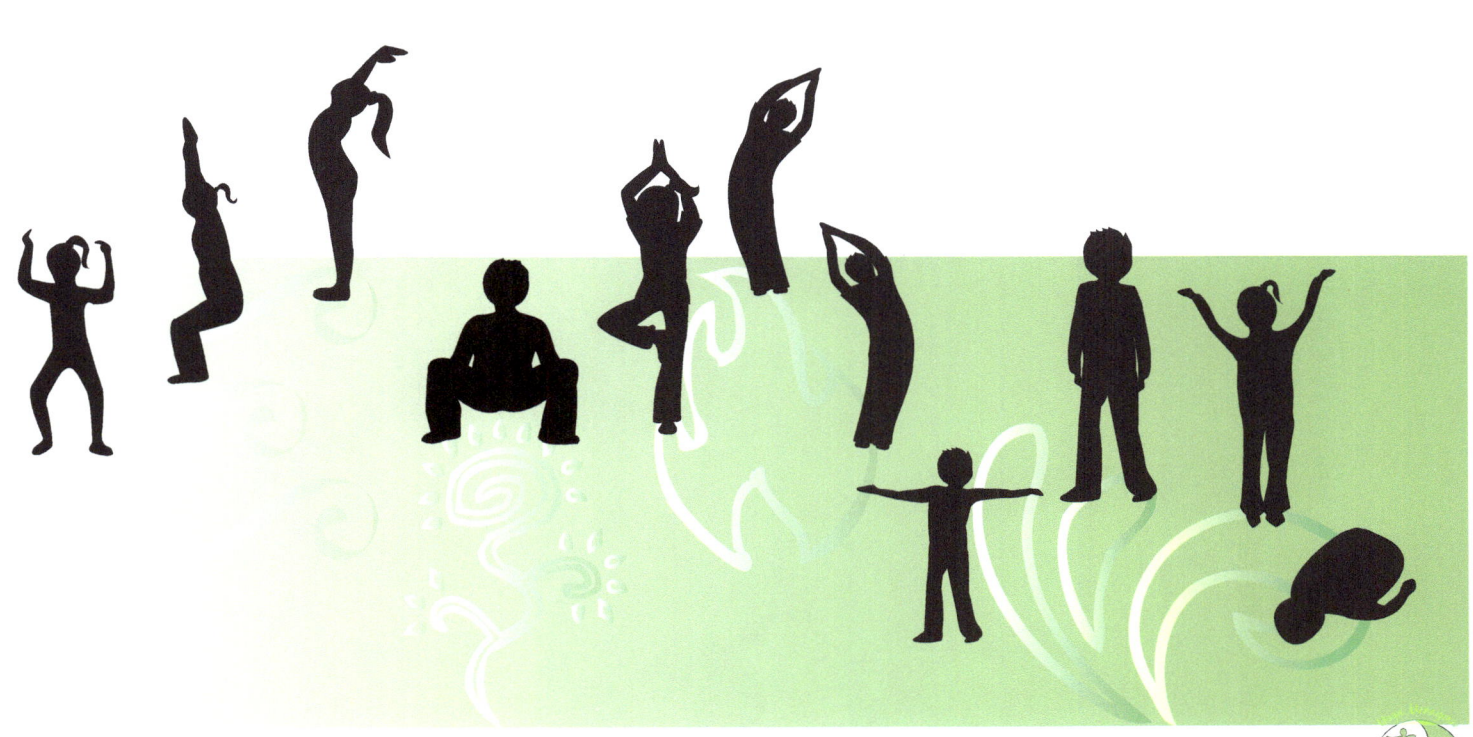

Mood Lifting
BALANCE

When I need to lift my mood;	*Bird – Right*
I balance until I feel good.	
I pretend that I'm a bird;	*Bird – Left*
Flying high above the herd.	
Then a flamingo with one leg up;	*Flamingo - Right*
This stretch helps me to perk up.	*Flamingo - Left*
Sometimes, I pretend I'm a tree;	*Tree - Right*
Doing this brings peace to me.	*Tree - Left*
The ladybug is so very small;	*Ladybug*
But she's the calmest one of all.	
It's time to get in our little boat;	*Boat*
Get rocked around and ready to float.	*Armadillo*
Lift up to be a candlestick;	*Candlestick*
Hurry, catch your balance quick!	
Push up flat to be a table;	*Table*
Lift one arm and leg if you are able.	*Lift*
On your side to be a rainbow;	*Rainbow*
Lift up high and then let go.	
Over to plank – just like a log;	*Plank*
Push up strong to be a dog.	*Down Dog*
Balancing always lifts my mood;	*Triangle*
It really helps me to feel good.	*Mountain*

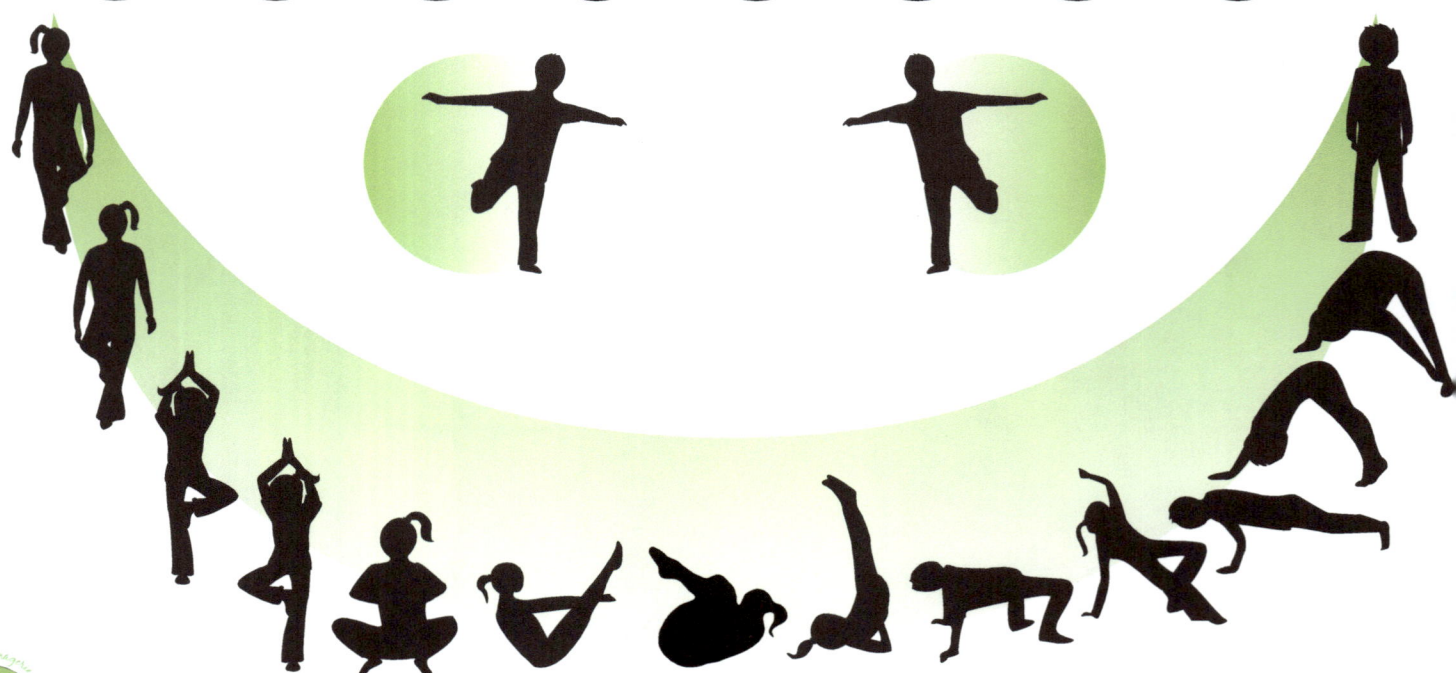

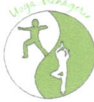

Adventure
THROUGH THE FOREST

In the forest, with the tallest trees,	*Tree*
The ladybugs want to play with me.	*Ladybug*
The spider crawls by, so he can make way;	*Spider*
For the big green turtle to come out and play.	*Turtle*
The bear looks left, the bear looks right,	*Bear – left/right*
He roars to his friends with all of his might.	*Bear – center*
Butterfly, come fly away with me,	*Butterfly*
Let's soar up to the highest tree.	*Staff*
The deer looks back. What does she see?	*Deer – right*
All the friends that came to play with me!	*Deer – left*
The cat lifts his head up so high,	*Cat Tilt-Up*
Then hides it again; because sometimes he's shy.	*Cat Tilt- Down*
Little tiny buzzing bee,	*Bee 1*
Come play the day away with me.	*Bee 2*

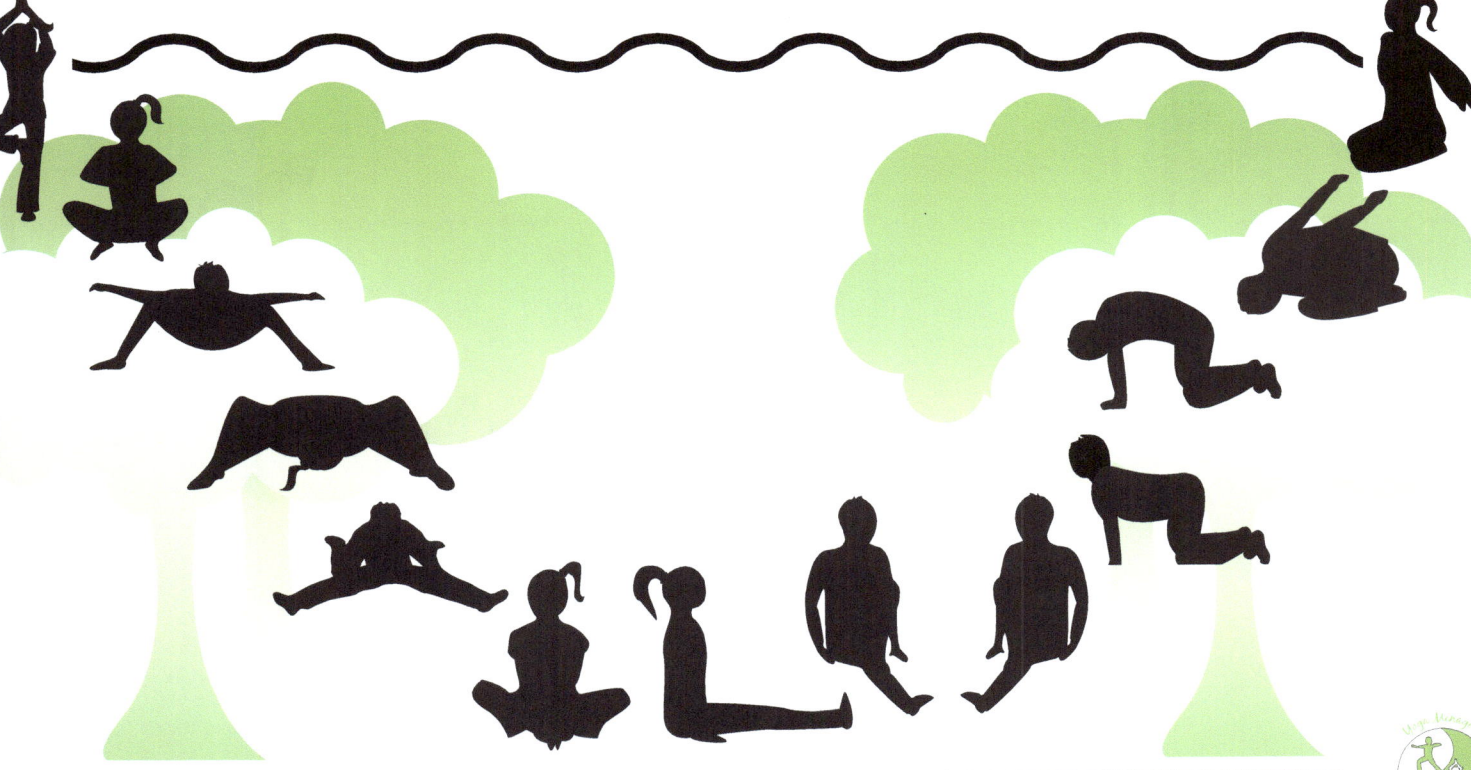

Snow Adventure

Snowflakes are falling, winter is here; This is the very best time of the year.	*Star/Snowflake Palm Press*
Wrap up tight and keep yourself warm; Get ready for the big snowstorm.	*Half Boat*
We'll gather the snow up from the ground; And build a snowman nice and round.	*Reach and scoop Snowman / 8*
Then we'll go sledding down a great big hill; Sliding so fast is a wintery thrill.	*Half Boat*
Let's make a giant snowball, And roll it all around; Playing in the snow is the coolest fun around.	*Snowball/Tuck in Armadillo Star / Snowflake*

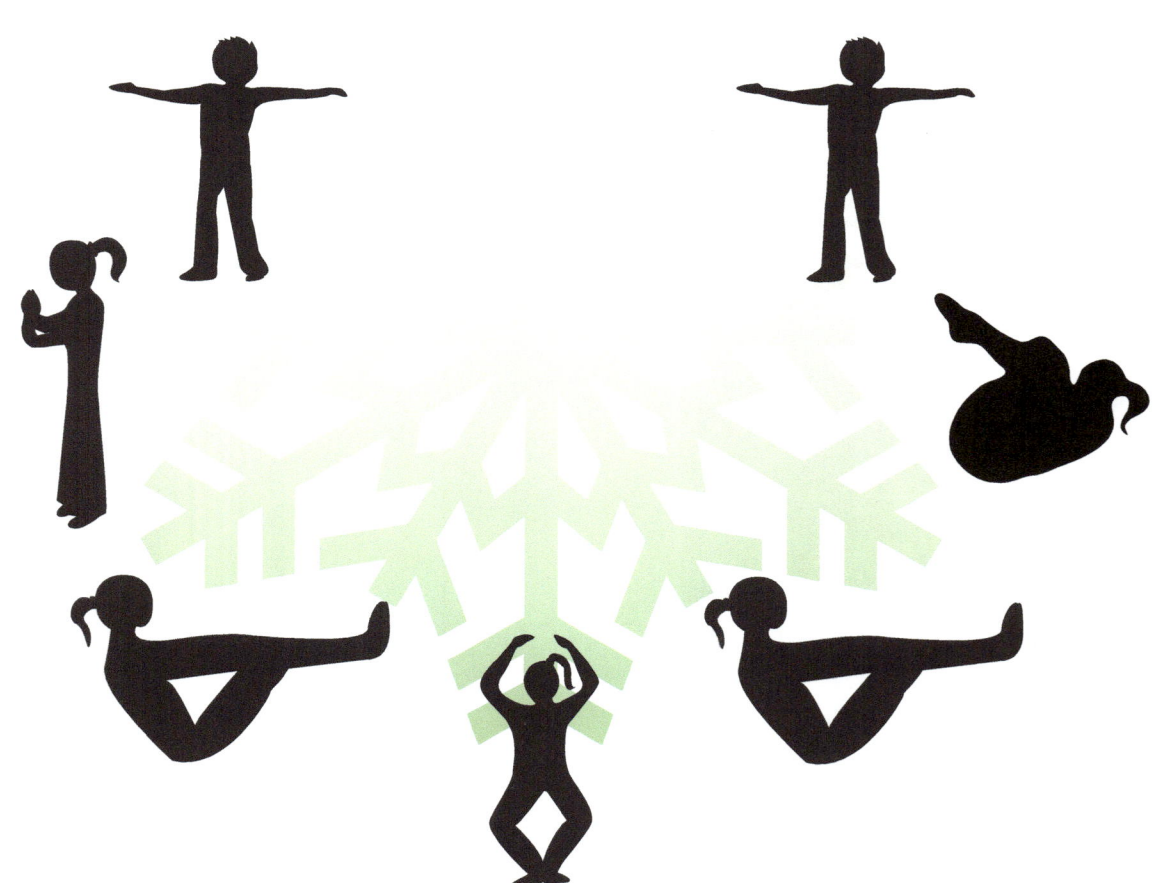

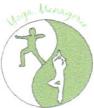

Butterfly's Adventure

Butterfly, butterfly, up in the sky;
Butterfly, butterfly, soaring so high.
Butterfly, butterfly, swoop down low;
Smell the flowers as you go.

Butterfly
Bear
Butterfly
Bend Forward

Butterfly, butterfly, come sit with me;
It's the turtle by this tree.
Sometimes turtle plays with her
friend the spider;
And sometimes she doesn't like anyone
beside her.

Butterfly
Turtle
Spider

Turtle-tuck head

Butterfly, butterfly, up in the sky;
Butterfly, butterfly, soaring so high.
Butterfly, butterfly, swoop down low;
Smell the flowers as you go.

Butterfly
Bear
Butterfly
Bend Forward

Butterfly, butterfly, fly with me;
Butterfly, butterfly, who do you see?
It's an owl that we've found;
Watch him twist himself around.
Butterfly, butterfly, please come here;
In the meadow is the little deer.
The little deer loves to jump and play;
He runs about all thru the day.

Butterfly
Circle Forward
Owl - Right
Owl – Left
Butterfly
Deer
Deer - Right
Deer - Left

Butterfly, butterfly, up in the sky;
Butterfly, butterfly, soaring so high.
Butterfly, butterfly, swoop down low;
Smell the flowers as you go.

Butterfly
Bear
Butterfly
Bend Forward

Butterfly, butterfly, look over there;
Let's go visit the big brown bear.
He claws about and growls some more;
Then lets out a mighty roar.
Now butterfly's been to see all her friends;
Tomorrow she will do it again.

Butterfly
Bear - Right
Bear - Left
Bear - Center
Butterfly
Bear

Butterfly, butterfly, up in the sky;
Butterfly, butterfly, soaring so high.
Butterfly, butterfly, swoop down low;
Smell the flowers as you go.

Butterfly
Bear
Butterfly
Bend Forward

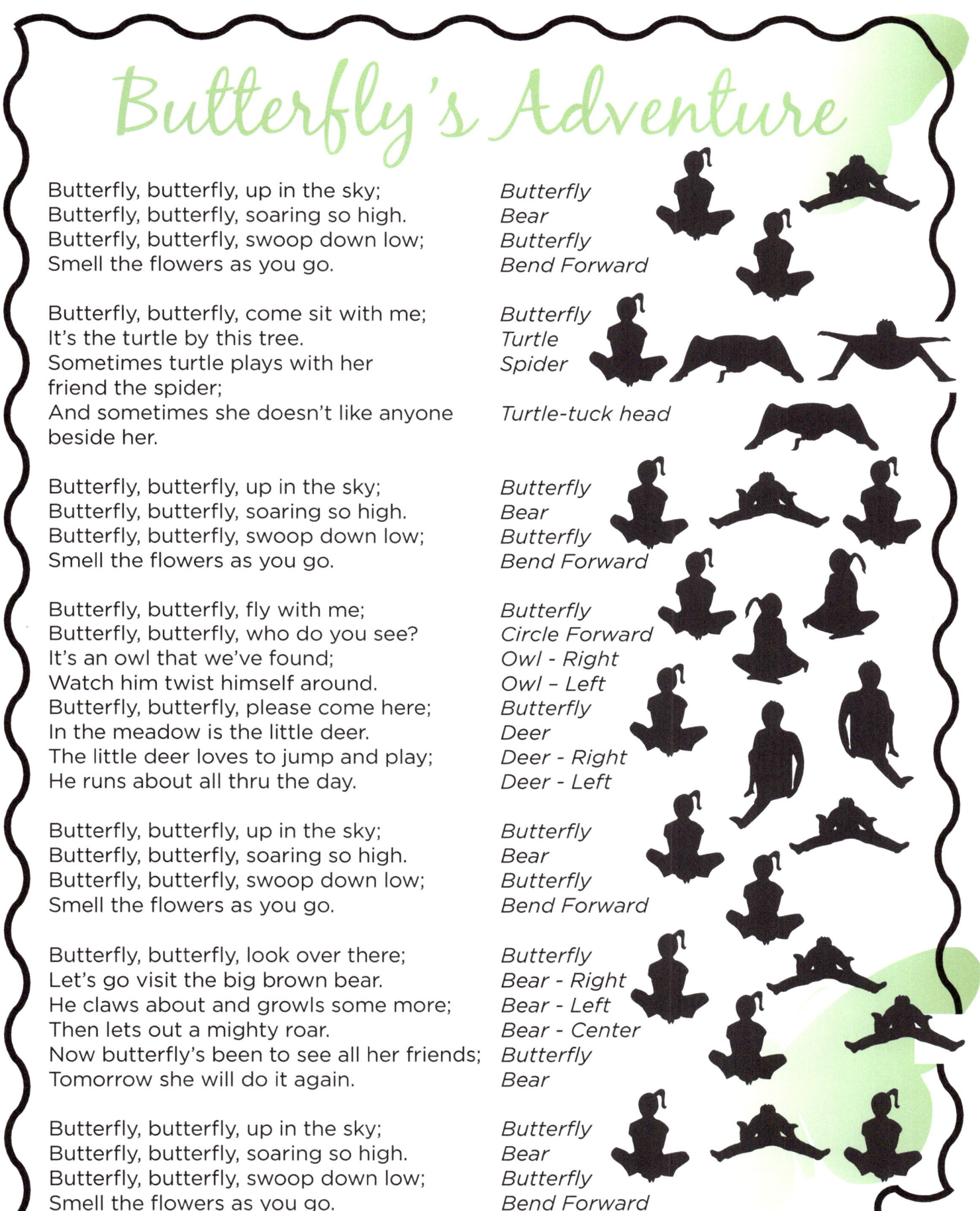

ADVENTURES IN
KIDS YOGA
Chapter Three

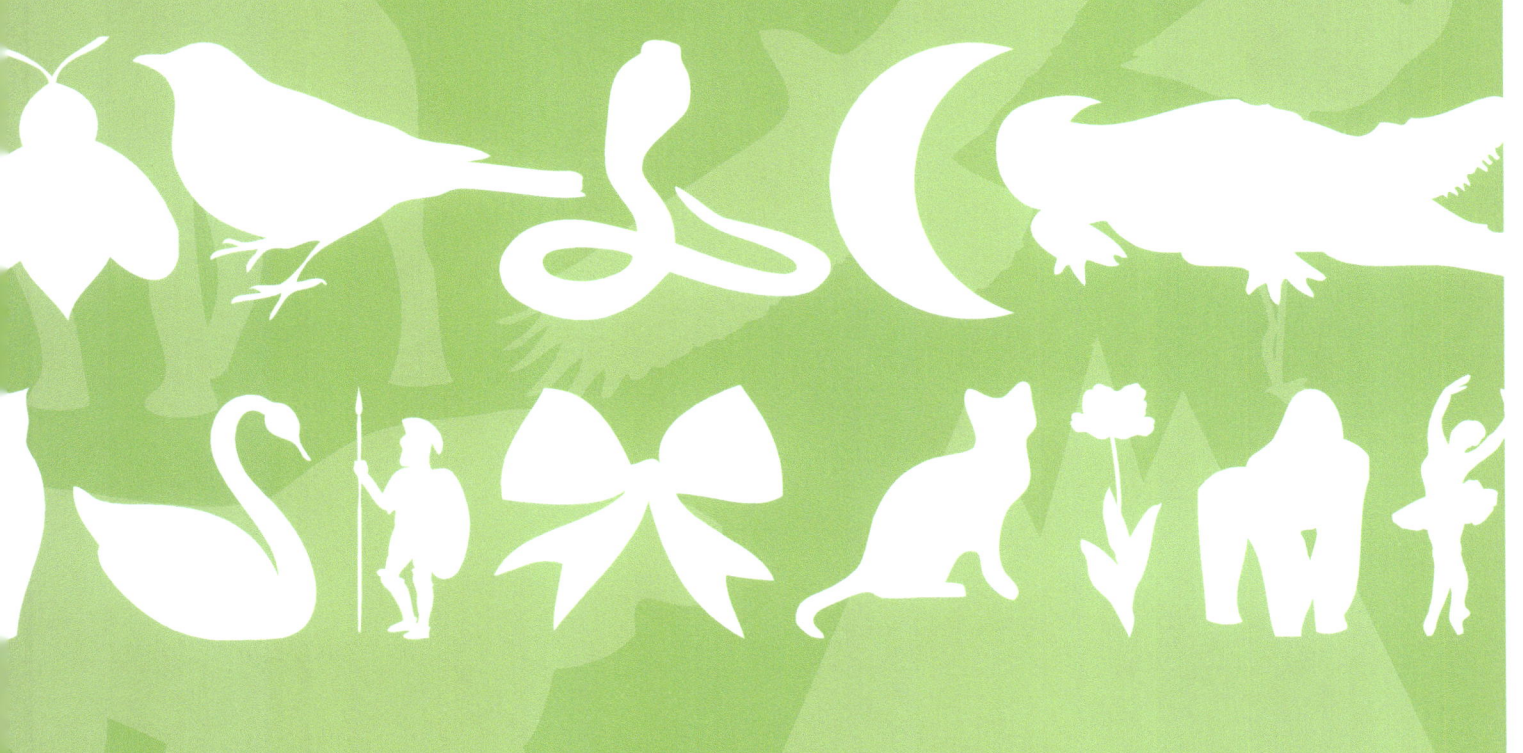

Adventure in the Park

When the sun rises up to the middle of the sky,	*Sun*
And the fluffy clouds go floating by.	*Reach side to side*
Meet me by the old oak tree;	*Tree*
I've made a picnic for you and me	*Arms up*
The ladybugs come out to play	*Ladybug*
On this bright and sunny day.	*Sun*
At the pond the frogs all hop,	*Frog*
Ducks waddle around; the fun never stops.	*Duck 1*
The giant tortoise is my friend;	*Turtle*
When he's scared he hides his head	
The wise old owl can twist and bend;	*Owl – right*
Reach around and twist again.	*Owl – left*
Beautiful Butterflies flutter by with a zoom,	*Butterfly*
Pollinating the flowers and making them bloom	*Flower*
Behind the rock I think I see;	*Rock*
A slithering snake looking back at me.	*Cobra*
There's a little cat tucked in for nap,	*Cat Tilts – down*
She lifts her head and meows like that.	*Cat Tilts – up*
The great big dog stretches up high,	*Down Dog*
Lifts his head and barks at the sky.	*Lift Head*
When the moon rises high over our heads;	*Crescent Moon-Right*
It's time to go home and get ready for bed.	*Crescent Moon-Left*
See the stars shining bright;	*Star*
Make a wish and say "Good Night."	*Wiggle Fingers*

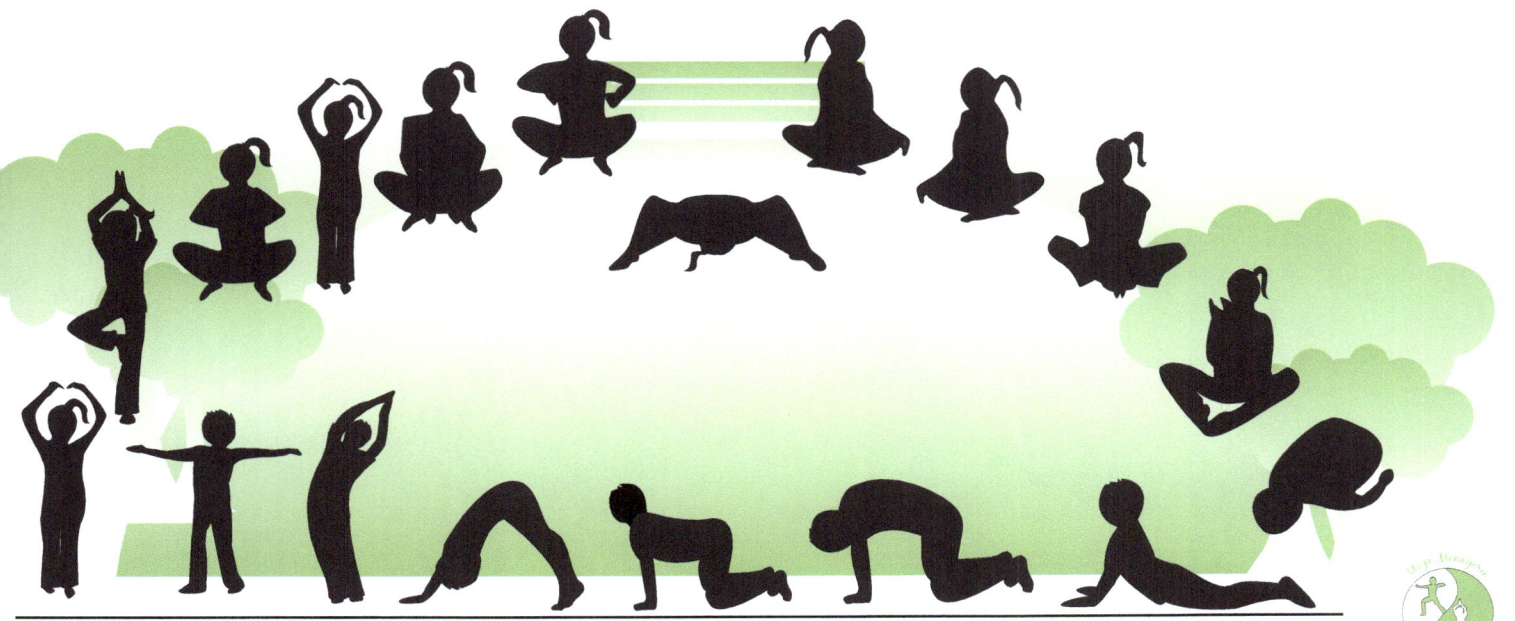

Outback Adventure

Hopping around like a kangaroo;	*Hop*
Adventuring thru the outback too.	
The eagles soar over the mountaintops;	*Eagle – Right*
Over the desert and Ayer's Rock.	*Eagle – Left*
The koala bear likes to nap in the trees;	*Bear – R & L*
If he isn't sleeping, he's eating leaves.	*Bear – Center*
Some animals in the outback can be scary;	
Here spiders are big and really hairy.	*Spider*
The snakes are scaly; they will give you a fright;	*Cobra*
And watch out for the crocodile - he bites!	*Crocodile*
In the bush there are dingoes – the wild dogs;	*Down Dog*
And in the rainforest hops the green tree frogs.	*Frog*
Kookaburra's a bird that sits high in the tree;	*Bird – Right*
It sounds like he's laughing with me.	*Bird – Left*
From the desert to the seashore;	*Star*
The outback's a wild place to explore.	*Mountain*

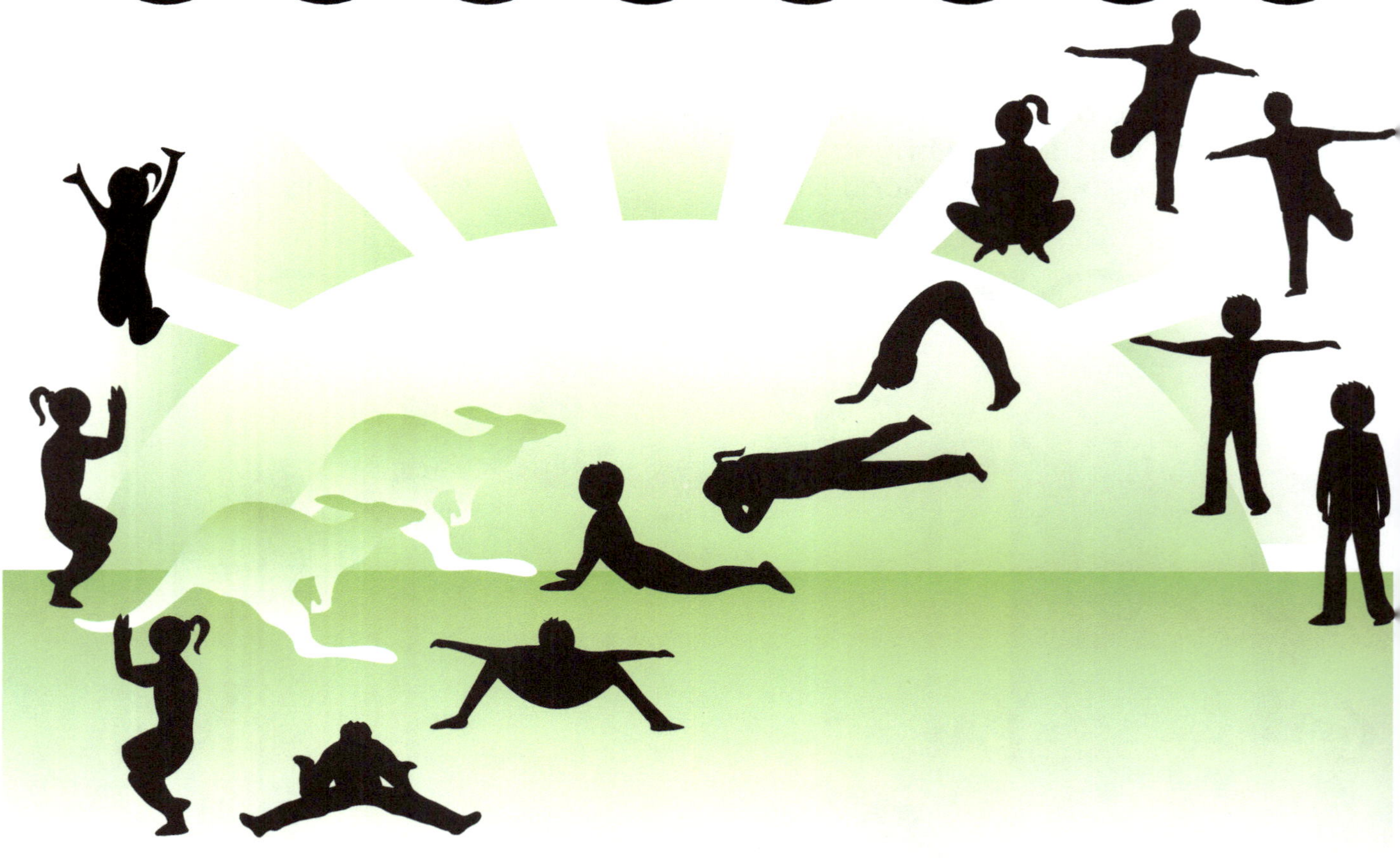

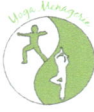

Submarine Adventure

Come along and explore with me;	*Boat*
In a submarine under the sea.	
Follow the current – Hurry along!	*Mermaid – Right*
Listen for the mermaid's song!	
There she goes– stay on her trail.	*Mermaid – Left*
Watch her flip her fishy tail.	
The stingray goes on sailing by;	*Stingray*
Spreading his fins like he can fly.	
The seal leads us along the way;	*Seal*
On the adventure we're having today.	
As our sub sinks down, it's getting dark...	*Shark*
Better watch out for the Shark!	
Hurry - Let's find a place to hide;	*Rock*
How about by the mountainside.	*Mountain*
This mountain's shaking, it's about to blow;	*Mountain-raise hands*
It's an underwater volcano!	*Volcano*
We've sailed our sub on all the waves;	*Warrior 2*
Exploring the reefs & all the caves.	*Warrior 3*
Discovering the ocean was super cool;	*Circle Around*
But next time – let's go to the pool!	*Mountain*

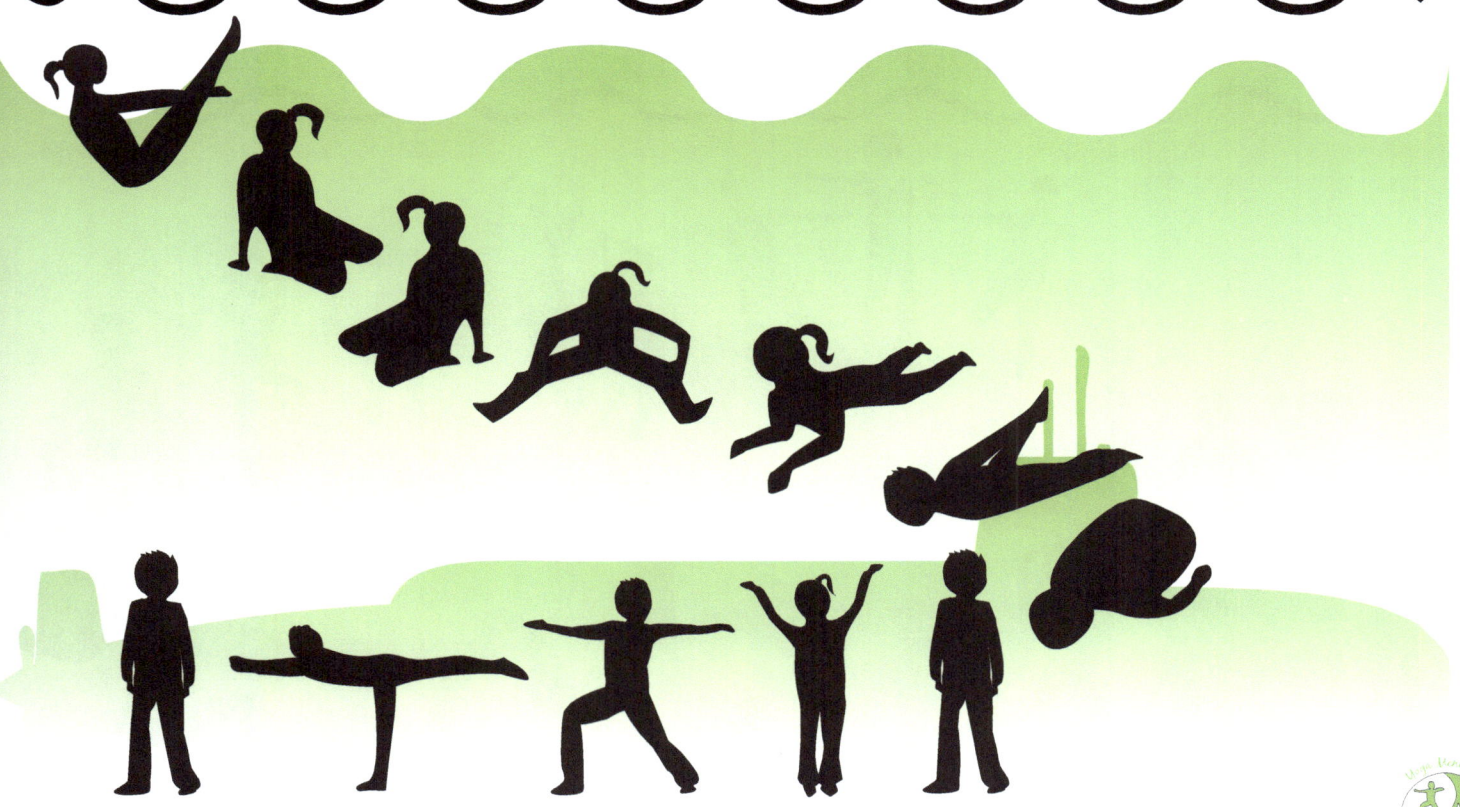

Adventure into Space

Get ready now and take your place;	*Mountain -hands*
Aboard our rocket to outer space.	*Palm Press-up*
The countdown is starting, get ready to take off;	*Arms down to side*
3... 2... 1... Blast Off!	*Palm Press-up*
Cruising like a comet thru the stars	*Bird - Star*
We're moving so fast... it doesn't seem far.	*Bird-reverse*
Around the Moon and past the sun,	*Crescent Moon/Sun*
Exploring the galaxy is really fun.	*Circle around*
At the North Star go Left,	*Star*
At the Big Dipper go Right,	*Tree*
The Asteroid Belt... will soon be in sight.	*Asteroid-Squat*
We'll roll thru and get tossed around;	*Armadillo/ roll to back*
The crab nebula is next to be found.	*Crab*
A meteor is a kind of space rock,	*Rock-meteor*
Drifting thru the universe...Where will it stop?	*Roll to Rock*
Constellations are pictures hidden in the sky,	
This one looks like a giant dog floating by.	*Down Dog*
The pictures are made by connecting the stars;	*Star*
Here is the archer ...shooting his arrow so far.	*Archer*
Soaring a rocket thru outer space was fun;	*Diving Dolphin*
But back to Earth we go...	*Open Hero*
Our adventure is done!	*Mountain*

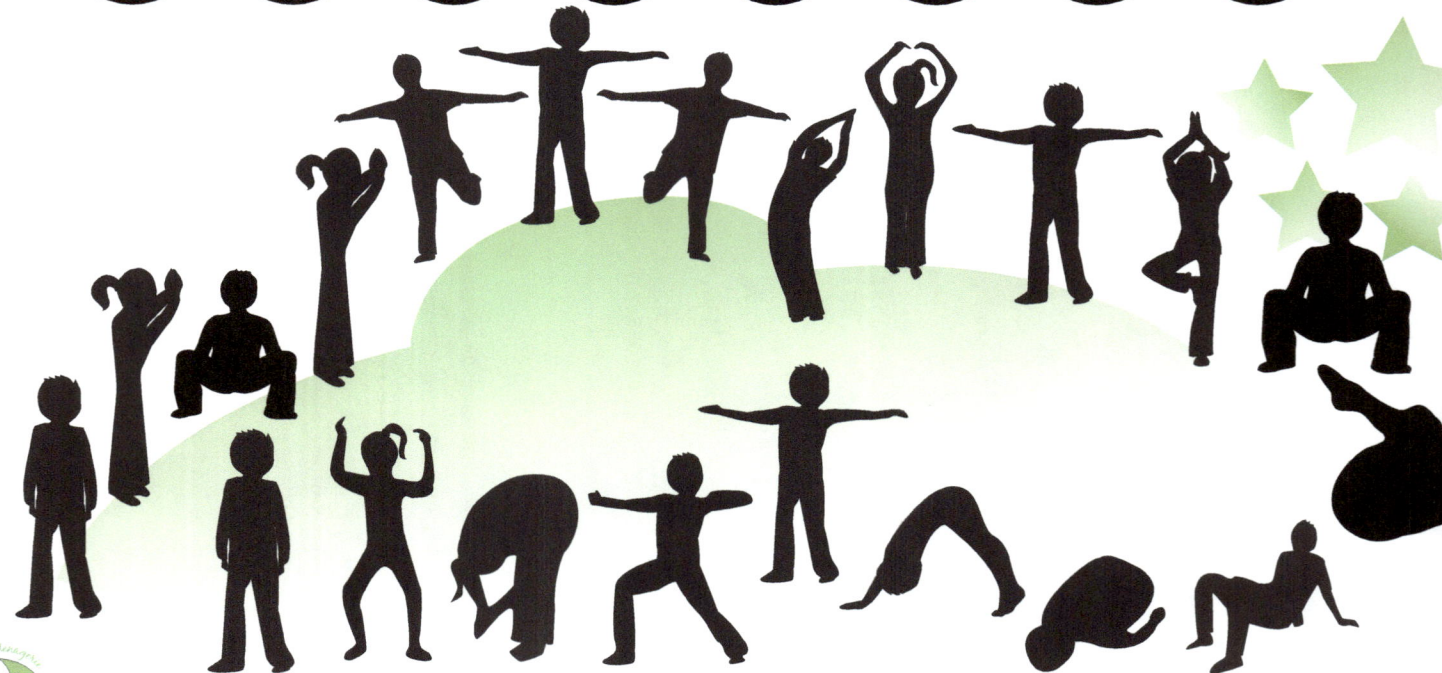

ADVENTURES IN KIDS YOGA

Chapter Four

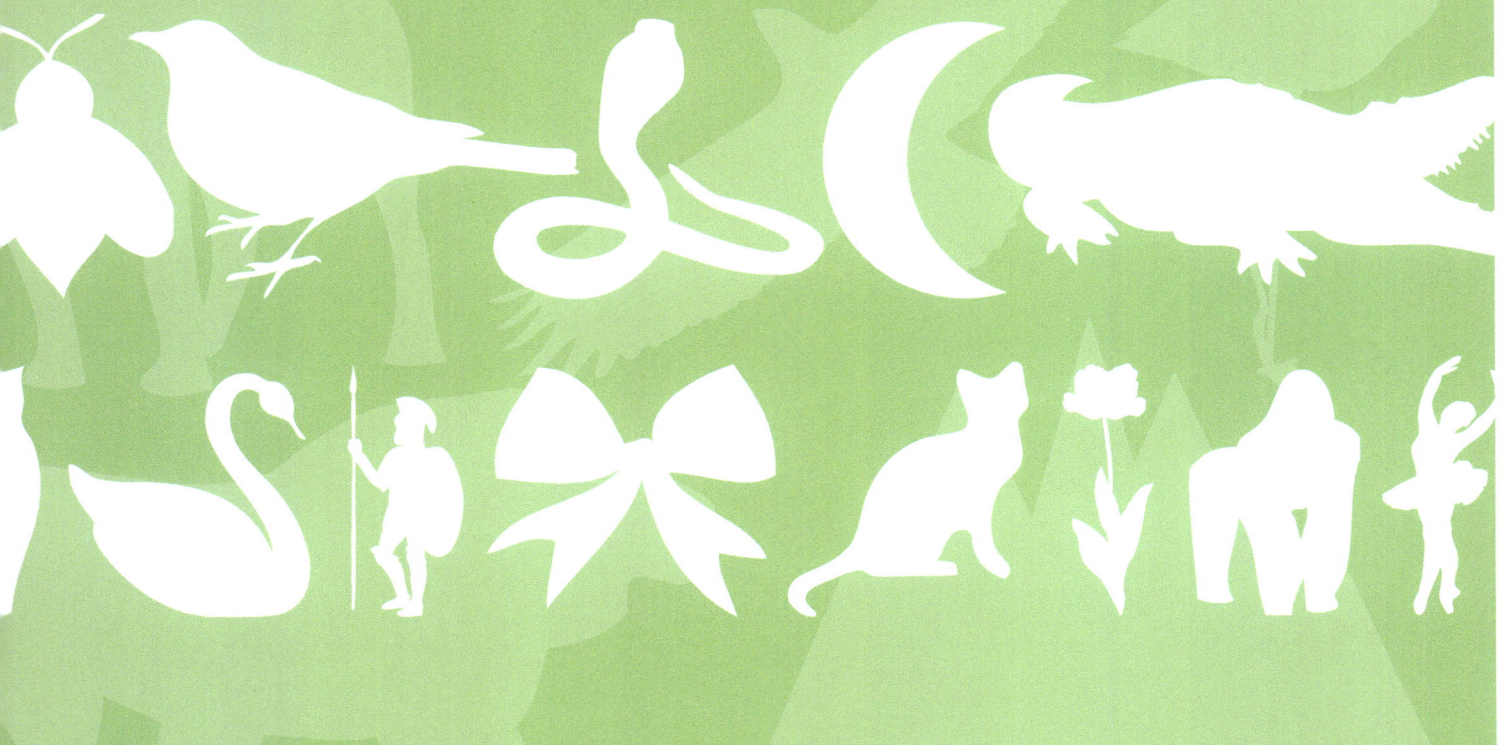

Road Trip Adventure

Its road trip time! Get in the car!	*Car – Boat*
We're going really, really far.	
Buckle up and get comfy as can be,	*Washing Machine*
Let's look out the window & see what we can see.	*Look out*
Look and see the beautiful flowers;	*Flower*
I could sit and watch for hours.	
There a toad hops along his way.	*Frog*
He jumps around and plays all day.	
The wild horses gallop so free;	*Horse*
Running this way and that among the trees.	
The Eagle flies high – Where will he stop?	*Eagle*
On the highest mountaintop.	*Mountain*
The mountain is full of beautiful trees;	*Tree*
With their leaves swaying in the breeze.	
There's a beautiful waterfall	*Waterfall*
Flowing into the river;	*Diving Dolphin*
If you were to jump in you'd get quite a shiver.	*Washing Machine*
The hawks are circling in the sky;	*Bird*
We see them swoop as we drive by.	
I love to watch the animals play;	*Mountain*
And look at the view along the way	*Circle Around*
But don't be sad our adventure is done;	*Reach up*
Getting there is only half the fun.	*Squat down*
We've seen so many things here in the car.	*Car - Boat*
This road trip was the best by far.	

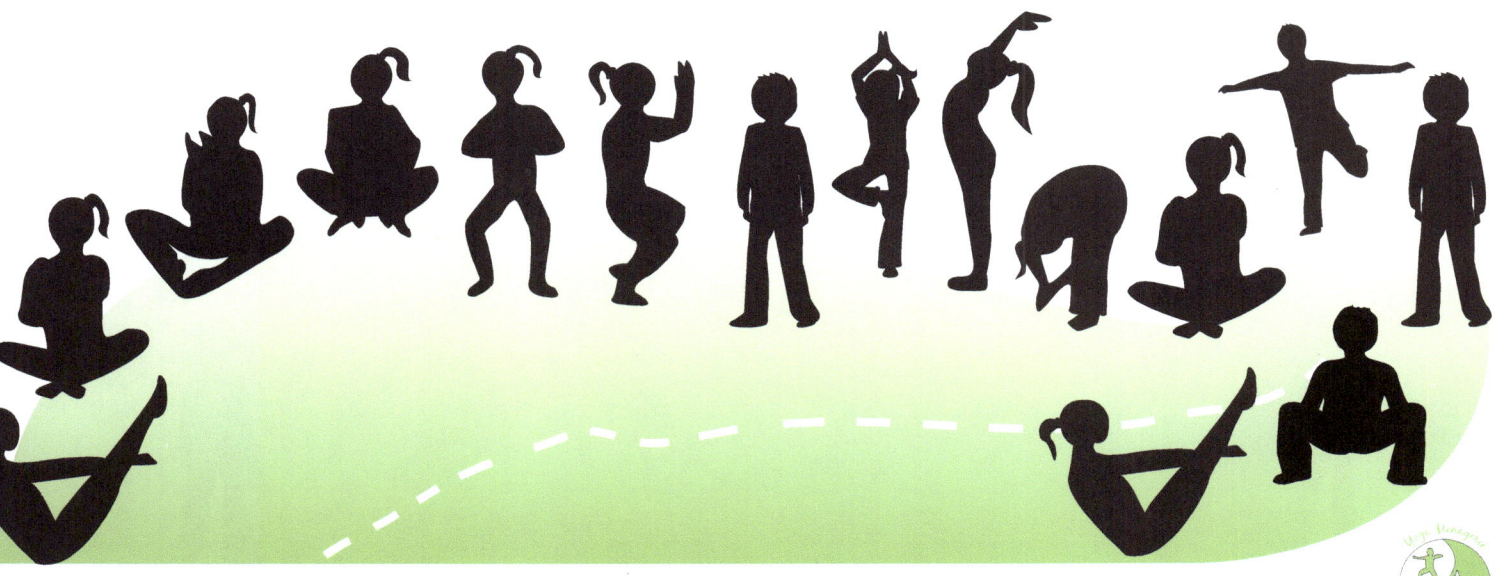

An Arctic Adventure

Up in the Arctic in the ice and snow.	*Mountain – arms up*
We're on an adventure – Here we go!	
The seals jump into the chilly sea;	*Seal - Diving Dolphin*
They look as happy as can be.	
There is the snow owl looking around;	*Owl – Right*
Watching his friends down on the ground.	*Owl – Left*
The polar bear is on the prowl;	*Bear – Reach Right*
Listen as he lets out a growl.	*Left Bear – Reach Center*
The reindeer prance along the snow;	*Deer-Right*
Putting on a magical show.	*Deer- Left*
Look at the iceberg floating by;	*Rock*
And the walrus looking up at the sky.	*Cobra or Seal*
There's a humpback whale swimming by;	*Whale*
He lifts his tail up to say "Hi."	
The Arctic fox is brave and bold;	*Fox - Down Dog*
He runs so fast he must be cold!	
At the top of the mountain you can see all about;	*Triangle*
The Arctic is the coolest place to chill out!	*Mountain*

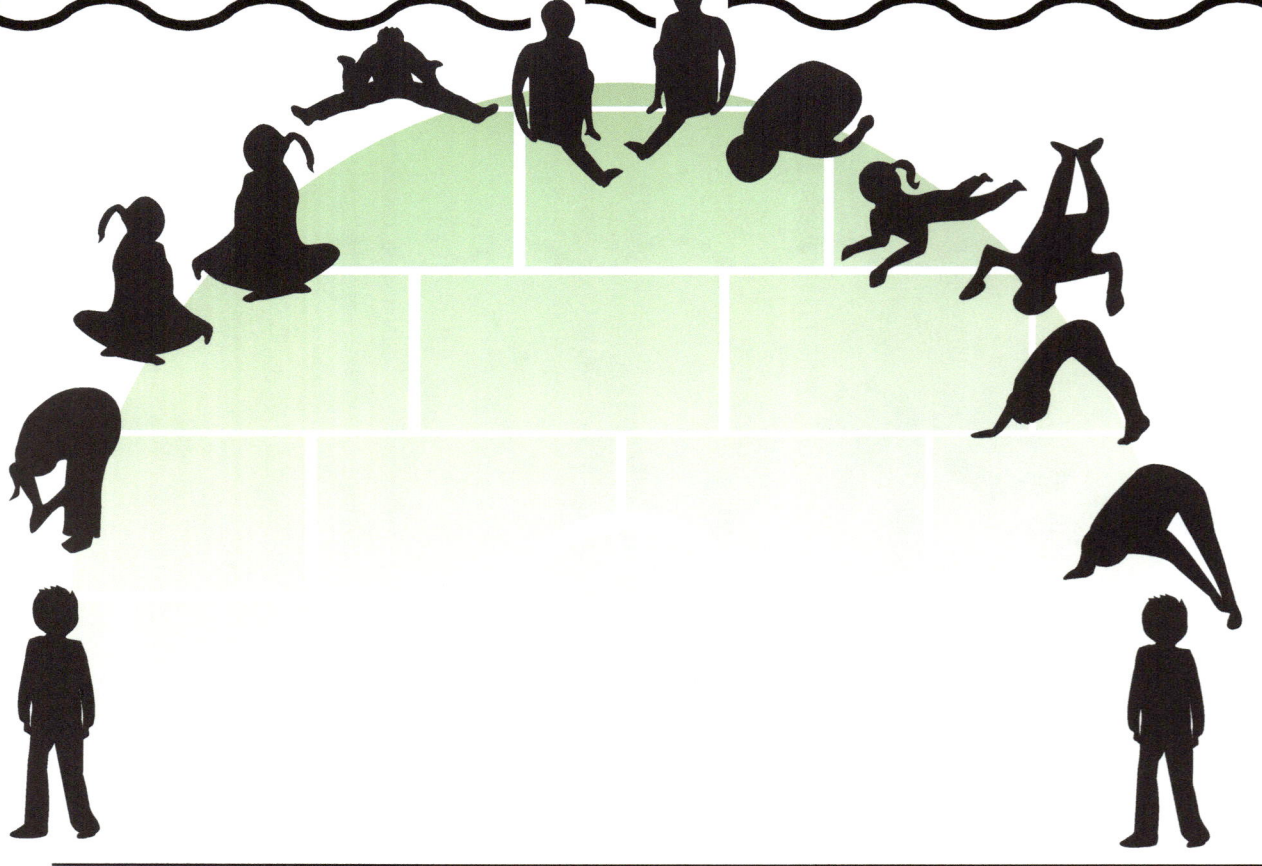

The Safari Adventure

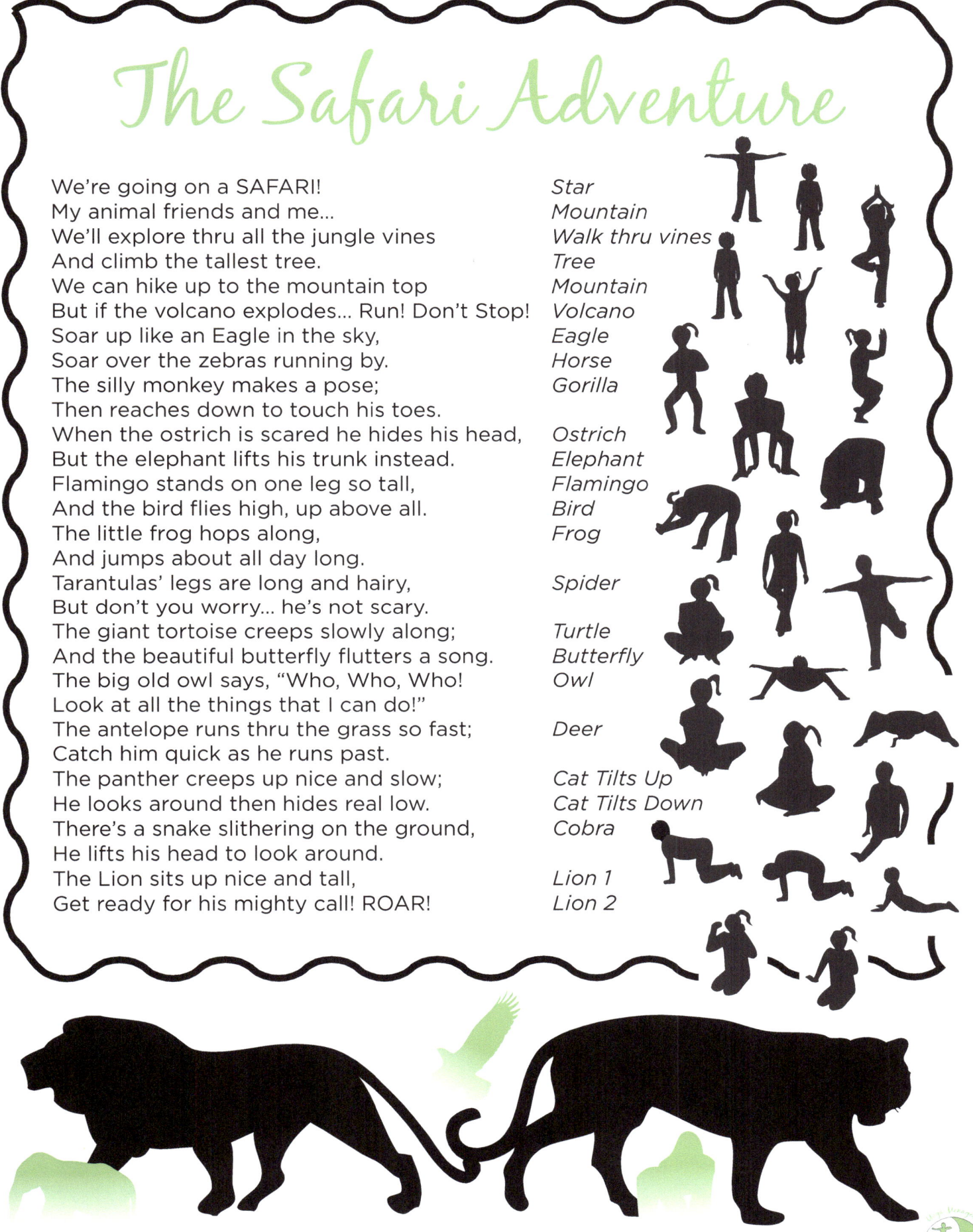

We're going on a SAFARI! — Star
My animal friends and me... — Mountain
We'll explore thru all the jungle vines — Walk thru vines
And climb the tallest tree. — Tree
We can hike up to the mountain top — Mountain
But if the volcano explodes... Run! Don't Stop! — Volcano
Soar up like an Eagle in the sky, — Eagle
Soar over the zebras running by. — Horse
The silly monkey makes a pose; — Gorilla
Then reaches down to touch his toes.
When the ostrich is scared he hides his head, — Ostrich
But the elephant lifts his trunk instead. — Elephant
Flamingo stands on one leg so tall, — Flamingo
And the bird flies high, up above all. — Bird
The little frog hops along, — Frog
And jumps about all day long.
Tarantulas' legs are long and hairy, — Spider
But don't you worry... he's not scary.
The giant tortoise creeps slowly along; — Turtle
And the beautiful butterfly flutters a song. — Butterfly
The big old owl says, "Who, Who, Who! — Owl
Look at all the things that I can do!"
The antelope runs thru the grass so fast; — Deer
Catch him quick as he runs past.
The panther creeps up nice and slow; — Cat Tilts Up
He looks around then hides real low. — Cat Tilts Down
There's a snake slithering on the ground, — Cobra
He lifts his head to look around.
The Lion sits up nice and tall, — Lion 1
Get ready for his mighty call! ROAR! — Lion 2

The Pirate's Adventure

A Pirate set out on the great blue sea,	*Hero*
To find out how strong he really could be.	*Arms flex, Hero*
He surfed on the waves, and sailed on the surf,	*Warrior 2*
He claimed the whole ocean as his home turf.	*Circle around*
He sailed by the sun, and followed the stars,	*Sun, Star*
Floating under the moon was his favorite by far.	*Crescent Moon*
His boat was the best, it never sank,	*Boat*
And all the bad guys had to walk the plank.	*Plank*
He was friends with the fish, even the shark.	*Shark*
His best friend was the sea serpent	*Cobra*
That came out after dark.	
He spotted an island, with palm trees so tall;	*Mountain, Palm Tree*
That swayed in the wind, without a care at all.	*Palm Tree - Reverse*
He raced the dolphins to the edge of the shore;	*Diving Dolphin*
Then he grabbed his map for adventures & more.	*Open map*
It said to hop like a frog,	*Frog*
And swim like a sea horse,	*Horse*
Then to fly like a bird, which is the best of course!	*Eagle or Bird*
He zigged to the left and zagged to the right;	*Triangle – left/right*
He searched for the "X" with all of his might.	*X - Star*
The clues led to a waterfall,	*Waterfall*
Then mermaids at a lagoon.	*Mermaid -right*
He knew that he'd find the treasure soon.	*Mermaid -left*
The clams snapped their shells,	*Clam*
And the crabs crawled by;	*Crab*
And a rainbow reached up and over the sky.	*Rainbow*
At the edge of the rainbow,	*Tuck*
There was an "X" on the land;	*X- Star*
It's time to start digging	*Triangle – Right*
And search thru the sand.	*Triangle - Left*
He shoveled and dug, and shoveled and dug;	*Center Reach*
Then he pulled on the chest and gave a great tug.	*Pull to hips*
"The Treasure ", he said. "Yo Ho Ho! It's been	*Reach up*
Found! I'm going to share it,	*Reach out and down*
With the best friends around".	
Then he got back in his boat,	*Boat- half*
It rocked side to side;	*Rock – side to side*
And he rowed out to sea, and sailed with	*Boat – full*
the tide.	

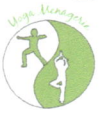

Halloween Adventure

When the moon is full, it's a spooky sight,	*Crescent Moon*
You know it must be Halloween night.	*X*
By the light of the stars what do you see?	*Star*
Lots of big old spooky trees...	*Tree*
Up in that tree is a big black cat.	*Cat Tilt -up*
He screeches' and hisses and meows like that.	*Cat Tilt - down*
Do you see the creepy spider?	*Spider - arms*
See him stretch his legs out wider.	*Spider – arms/legs*
On the fence is a wise old owl,	*Owl – right*
Looking around, he's on the prowl.	*Owl - left*
The big and hairy werewolf growls,	*Werewolf-down dog*
And then let's out a mighty howl.	*Lift head*
The goblins and ghouls are quite a sight	*Goblins/ghoul-lion*
Trying to give you a Halloween fright!	*Repeat*
Oh No! They chased us to the ridge;	*Roll to back*
Let's hurry across the old trolls' bridge.	*Bridge*
It's led us to the pumpkin patch;	*Roll to rock*
To find our perfect Halloween match.	*Wrap arms*
The bats soar up into the sky,	*Bat*
With the vampires and ghosts that are floating by.	*Cover face w/ arm-Star*
Our spooky adventure can't be beat;	*Squat*
But now it's time to say "trick or treat"	*Jump to Star*

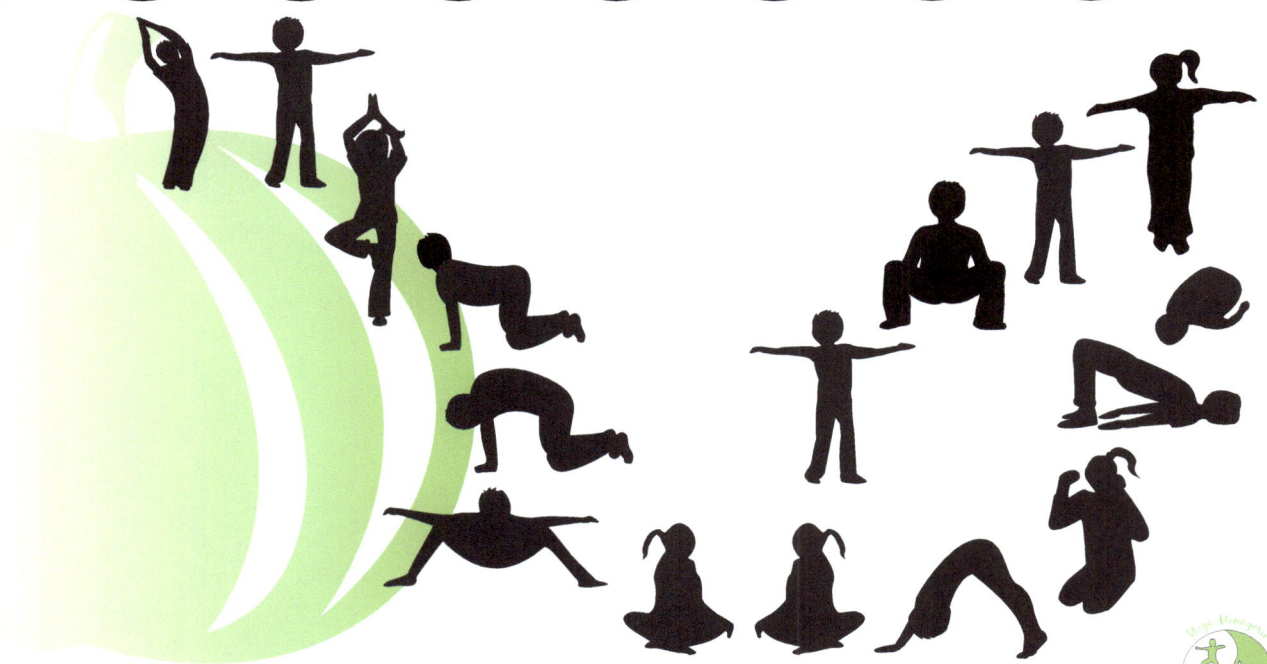

ADVENTURES IN KIDS YOGA

Chapter Five

A COLLECTION OF BREATHING TECHNIQUES AND SEQUENCES

Breathing Techniques

Breathing Techniques are an essential and fundamental part of all yoga practices. They help to cultivate numerous self-regulating and self-soothing skills. Proper breathing can help to reduce and manage stress by calming the parasympathetic nervous system and improving relaxation skills. However, breathing techniques can also be used to increase alertness, focus and energy.

Breathing Techniques and the proper use of breathe are a key aspect to all well-rounded yoga practices but they are also a self-empowering and valuable life skill that can be applied to every situation encountered on a daily basis. Proper breathing can help to shift the attitude and gain emotional, mental and physical stability. The following collection is a kid and family friendly version of the yoga breathing techniques. Each sequence is inspired by the pranayama breathing techniques.

NOTEWORTHY INFO AND SUGGESTIONS ON BREATHING

A breathing cycle usually consists of 3 parts: inhaling, exhaling and retention (holding the breathe in). Most practices begin by exhaling all of the air out of the body.

THERE ARE 3 KEY ASPECTS OF BREATH CONTROL EXERCISES

PLACE – where the breathe is coming from or where the breathe is directed
TIME – duration of inhales and exhales
NUMBER - # of repetitions in the cycle

Suggestions: dim the lights, use soft music, place hands on belly and chest and feel where breathe is coming from.

Try using objects to demonstrate and experiment with breathe: Pinwheels, straws or various sizes, feathers, balloons, balls, etc.

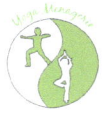

Sunflower Breaths

I started out small, as a tiny seed;   *Squat*
But watch me grow big and tall indeed.   *Bring arms out and up*

I reach out my leaves and follow the sun;   *Bring arms to the side*
Then close up my petals when I am done.   *Squat*

Mountain – Volcano
BREATHING SEQUENCE

A mountain stands up straight and sure;   *Mountain*
Its strength comes from its inner core.

Reaching up high and breathing in slow;   *Palm Press up*
Turn the mountain into a volcano.

It explodes with force and blows lava all around;   *Volcano*
It flows all the way unto the ground   *Mountain*

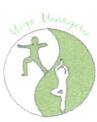

Tornado
BREATHING SEQUENCE

Spiraling like a tornado;	*Circle head*
Touching the clouds and the ground below.	*Add shoulders to circle*
Not too fast and not too slow-	*Add Rib cage to circle*
All the way around we go.	*Add stomach to circle*
	Butterfly – down

Octopus
BREATHING SEQUENCE

Giant Octopus under the sea; Come relax and breathe with me.	*Happy Baby*
With tentacles swaying wild and free; The tension floats away from me.	*Sway arms and legs side to side*
As the waves roll in and they roll out; I release the things I worry about.	*Bring arms and legs in* *Bring arms & legs out*
Stretching myself out so gracefully; I float along happy and free.	*Sand Angel* *Corpse*

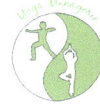

My Animal Friends
HELP ME WHEN I'M DOWN

When I'm mad I stomp around.
I stomp and stomp and stomp the ground;
Till I find my bunny friend...
We hop and hop and hop again.
Together we take a breath like a bunny,
123, 4 - 123, 4... isn't that funny.

Bunny Breath Sequence - 3 short inhales, 1 long exhale

Sometimes when I'm angry, I act bad and pout,
Then I ask my friend lion to come help me out.
I scrunch up my face and my hands before,
I let out a big, loud, mighty ROAR!

Lion's Breath Sequence
On inhale scrunch up face and hands and on exhale extend arms in front of you,
open hands and face

When I'm sad I ask the bee,
To sit beside and comfort me.
We buzz together to the count of four,
Sit up high – then touch the floor.

Bee Breath Sequence
Inhale for 4 counts then exhale for 4 counts - on the inhale sit up – arms behind
you like wings and on exhale buzz down to child's pose

My animal friends help me to calm down,
With bunny, lion and bee around;
I know I'll never get too mad,
Cause my animal friends make me really glad!

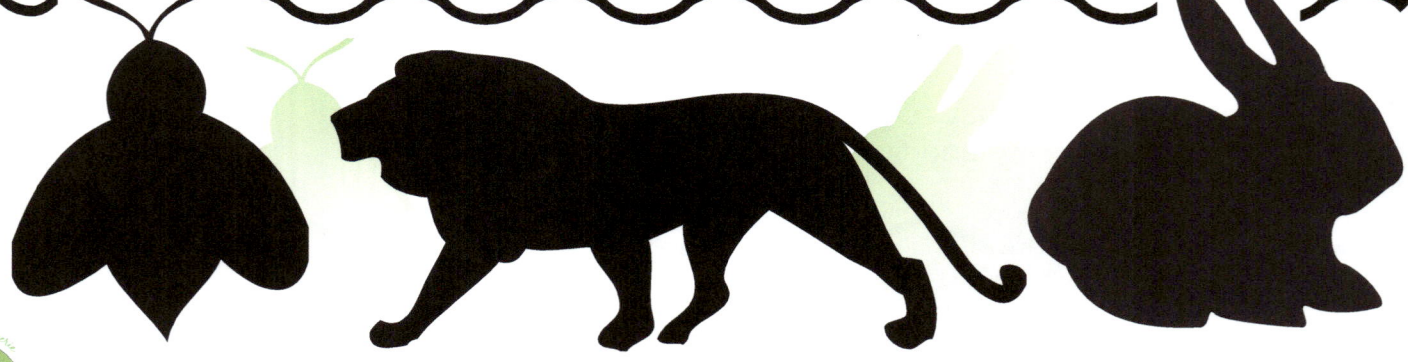

Bee Breathing

While inhaling - Rub hands together quickly
While exhaling – place hand over the eyes and nose making a buzzing sound

I rub my wings then cover my eyes;   *Bee 1*
So I can have a chance to look inside.

Making a special buzzing sound;   *Bee 2*
Lifting up and over to touch the ground.

Lion Breaths

Lion helps me get my feelings out;   *Sitting on the floor*
When I feel stressed – I give a shout.

First I squish my face and hands up tight;   *Lion 1*
And I inhale and focus with all my might.

When I exhale I open wide   *Lion 2*
My eyes, mouth and heart inside

Lion helps my true self soar;   *Return to sitting position chosen*
With all my heart – I let out a ROAR!   *above*

Dragon
BREATHING SEQUENCES

Fire Dragon

Inspired by Dirga / 3 part Breath

The fire dragon breathes in slow
And takes the air up thru its nose.

It holds it breathe a few seconds before;
Breathing fire with a mighty Roar!

Baby Fire Dragon

Inspired by Kapalabhati / Skull Shining / Breath of Fire

Baby Fire Dragon tucks its wings;
And looks within before it does anything.

Baby Fire Dragon sits up tall-
And spits out tiny fireballs!

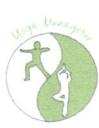

Smoke Dragon

Inspired by Sama Vritti / Equal Breathing

The Smoky Dragon uses its nose;
With equal breath is how it blows.

Inhaling gently and breathing slow;
Then exhaling smoke out of its nose.

Water Dragon

Inspired by Ujjayi/Ujay / Ocean Breath

The Water Dragon makes the sound of the ocean;
Using it's breathe to calm its emotion.

Sucking in the air with a "SSSS" sound;
Filling myself up with the peace that I've found.

Shooting out water from the back of the throat;
With a "HHHH" sound – its calmness I promote.

Ice Dragon

Inspired by Shitali / Cooling Breath

Ice Dragon rolls its tongue into a "U"
And uses its breathe to keep itself cool.

Thru the curl in the tongue cool air is inhaled;
Then out thru the nose all the heat is exhaled.

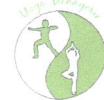

Yoga Journaling

Journaling or writing after you practice yoga is a great way to explore your ideas, create new ones and chart your yoga progress. Here are some questions to help you get started. You can use the blank pages here or get a whole other notebook just to contain your Yoga Ideas! (If your child isn't able to write or if you just need an outlet to open conversation than these questions can also be used to start a discussion in your class or home.)

WHICH POSE IS YOUR FAVORITE? WHY? _____

_____

_____

WHICH POSE IS THE HARDEST? WHY?_____

_____

_____

WHICH BREATHING EXERCISE IS YOUR FAVORITE? WHY? _____

_____

_____

WHICH BREATHING EXERCISE IS HARDEST? _____

_____

_____

WHICH POSE HELPS YOU TO FEEL THE BEST? WHY? _____

_____

_____

WHICH POSE IS MOST COMFORTABLE? WHY?_____

_____

_____

WHICH POSE HELPS YOU TO FEEL CALMEST? WHY?_____
_____
_____

WHICH POSE MAKES YOU FEEL THE MOST BALANCED? WHY?_____
_____
_____

WHICH POSE HELPS YOU FOCUS AND CONCENTRATE? WHY?_____
_____
_____

WHICH POSE "WAKES YOU UP" BEST? WHY?_____
_____
_____

WHICH POSE IS THE MOST RELAXING? WHY?_____
_____
_____

WHICH POSE HELPS YOU TO FEEL THE MOST STRETCHED OUT? WHY?_____
_____
_____

WHICH POSE HELPS YOU TO FEEL THE HAPPIEST? WHY?_____
_____
_____

WHICH POSE HELPS YOU TO OPEN UP TO NEW THINGS OR LET GO OF NEGATIVE THINGS?
WHY?_____
_____

WHICH POSE HELPS YOU TO PAY ATTENTION? WHY?_____
_____
_____

HICH POSE HELPS YOU TO BREATHE? WHY?_____

_____

_____

HICH POSE MAKES YOU FEEL SAFE? WHY?_____

_____

_____

HICH POSE TAKES THE MOST CONCENTRATION? WHY? _____

_____

_____

HEN DO YOU USE THE POSES IN YOUR DAILY LIFE?_____

_____

_____

OW DO YOU USE YOUR YOGA IDEAS IN YOUR LIFE?_____

_____

_____

HICH POSE OR SEQUENCE IS THE EASIEST? HARDEST? YOUR FAVORITE? ETC.? _____

_____

_____

OW IS THIS POSE AFFECTING YOUR ENERGY? (PHYSICALLY AND MENTALLY) _____

_____

_____

D THE BREATHING EXERCISE "QUIET YOUR MIND" OR "ACCELERATE" IT?_____

_____

_____

HICH SEQUENCE GIVES YOU THE MOST BENEFIT? THE BIGGEST BREATHS? _____

_____

_____

_____

WHICH OPENS AND STRENGTHENS YOUR LUNGS THE BEST? _____

_____

_____

WHAT EMOTIONS DOES THE SEQUENCE PROMOTE IN YOU? _____

_____

_____

DOES THE SEQUENCE STEADY THE MIND AND BODY?_____

_____

_____

CAN YOU FEEL THE RHYTHMS IN THE DIFFERENT BREATHS? _____

_____

_____

WHICH RHYTHM DO YOU LIKE THE BEST? _____

_____

_____

WHICH BREATHING SEQUENCE IS THE MOST USEFUL FOR YOU IN YOUR DAILY ACTIVITIES?

_____

_____

ADVENTURES IN
KIDS YOGA
Glossary

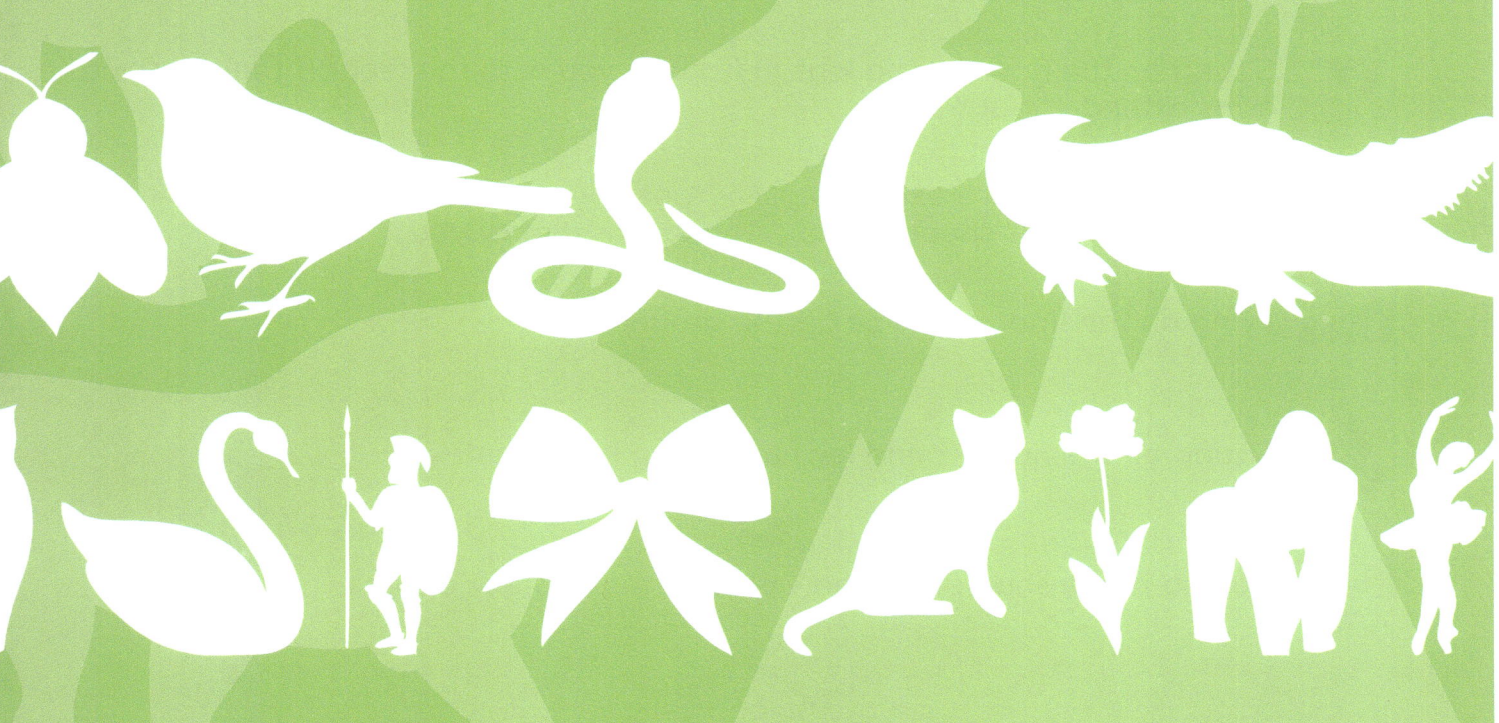

Glossary

ADVENTURES IN KIDS YOGA (BOOK ONE)

ARCHER
Standing with feet apart - one foot facing front - the other facing the side; extend the same arm as foot facing to the side and use the other to pull back a bow (bent arm - pull hand to shoulder)

ARMADILLO
Sitting on the floor - curl body into a ball and rock backward and forward

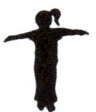
BAT
Stand feet together - arms extended out to the side - rise up on toes

BEAR
Sitting on the floor - extend legs out into a straddle and reach to the right, left and center

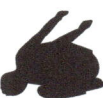
BEE
On knees- sit up and put arms behind you like wings then bring bend body forward to legs

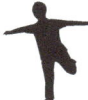
BIRD
Standing on one foot- lift the other leg behind you and bring your arms out to the side

BOAT - HALF
Sitting on the floor - bend legs in front of you with the feet off the floor and arms extended out front

BOAT - FULL
Sitting on the floor - extend legs in front of you - with legs off the ground, try to make a "V" shape- arms extended in front of you

BRIDGE
Lying on the floor - lift hips off the ground

BUTTERFLY
Sitting on the floor - bend legs and bring feet together

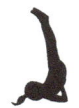
CANDLESTICK
Roll up into a shoulder stand - place arms on floor or hips

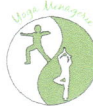

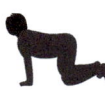
CAT TILTS UP
On the floor on hands and knees - arch back and look up

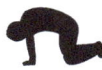
CAT TILTS DOWN
On knees - pull body back to sit on feet - arms extended and stretched out in front of you

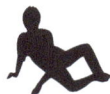
CLAM
Bend legs to your side and open your knees

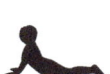
COBRA
Lying on stomach - straigten arms, lift chest and look up

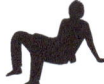
CRAB
On the floor - bend legs and place hands on floor and lift body slightly off the ground

CRESCENT MOON
Standing feet together- hands clasped overhead- reach over to the side

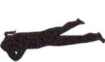
CROCODILE
On the floor lying on your stomach – extend feet out or arms out front and snap hands together like jaws

DIVING DOLPHIN
Standing feet together - hands in prayer - reach down to the floor and come back up in a wave motion

DEER
Sitting on the floor with legs extended in front of you - bend one leg into your chest and grab with your arms, then reverse

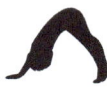
DOWN DOG
Place hands on the floor – feet apart- lift body into a "V" shape with the hips pointing up

DUCK
In squat - place arms bent to your sides and flap like wings

EAGLE
Cross one leg over the other and place arms to the side or behind you like wings and lean forward

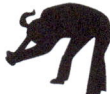
ELEPHANT
Standing feet spread apart - hands clasped together in front of you with arms extended out in front of you - bend forward then lift arms as trunk

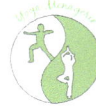

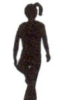
FLAMINGO
Standing on one leg – bend the other leg and place foot near knee or other foot

FLOWER
Sitting in butterfly - lift feet off ground or cup hands and lift up

FROG
Squat to floor and hop

GORILLA
Standing legs apart - bend forward and place hands or knees on floor

HERO
Standing with feet shoulder width apart or kneeling - hands on hips

HORSE
Standing legs apart - knees bent - hands in prayer - arms bent with elbows out to the side

LADYBUG
Squat - hands in palm press

LION
Kneeling – scrunch hands and face

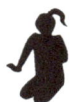
LION 2
Extend arms forward and unscrunch face - open mouth

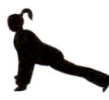
LIZARD
One leg bent – the other leg extended – place hands next to the foot on the floor

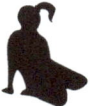
MERMAID
sitting on the floor - legs bent to your side

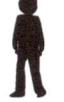
MOUNTAIN
Standing straight up - arms down to your sides

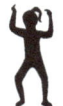
OPEN HERO
Standing legs apart – knees bent – arms extended out to the side and bent with hands pointing up

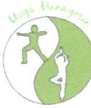

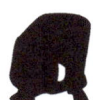
OSTRICH
Standing feet apart - cover head with arms and bend in half forward

OWL
Sitting on the floor- cross legs in front of you and reach one arm to the opposite side and twist then reverse

PALM PRESS
Hands together – fingertips pointing up

PALM TREE
Standing on one leg - the other leg bent with foot on knee - arms bent overhead - reverse arms and reverse legs

PEACOCK
Kneeling on one knee or lunge - extend arms behind you and lift up

PIGEON
On the floor - one leg extended behind you the other bent in front of you

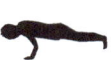
PLANK
Down on the floor – extend legs out behind you or bend knees on the ground - place hands in front of you on the floor and lift body off floor

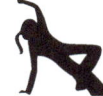
RAINBOW
On the floor facing the side - one leg straight with the other bent - lift hips off the ground - lift arm from side to your head and back down

ROCK - CHILD'S POSE
Kneeling on the floor lie chest on knees

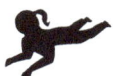
SEAL
Laying on your stomach - lift to elbows and lift your head up

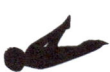
SHARK
Lying on the floor - clasp hands behind you and lift up to create a fin

SQUAT
Legs bend with hands touching the floor

SPIDER
In squat or on the floor with legs bent - arms extended out the side

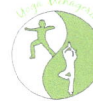

STAFF
Sitting on the floor - extend legs out in front of you

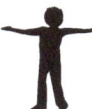
STAR
Standing feet apart with arms extended out to the side

STINGRAY
Sitting on the floor - open legs to a straddle and rach right, left and center

SUN
Standing feet together - round arms over head

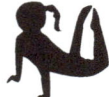
SWAN
On the floor lying on your stomach – lift feet up and roll head back

TREE
Standing on one leg - bend the other leg and bring the foot to touch the knee - hands in prayer

TRIANGLE
Standing feet apart – bend forward and touch your toes- right, left and center

TURTLE
Sitting on the floor - legs bent out the side - place arms under your knees and hands behind feet then tuck head down

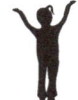
VOLCANO
Standing in mountain pose - hands in prayer - lift hands over head then open them and bring arms down to your sides

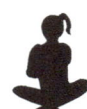
WASHING MACHINE
Cross arms around body and twist

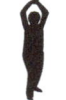
WARRIOR 1
Standing with leg straight with foot facing the side – other leg placed in front slightly bent- clasp hands and raise overhead

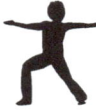
WARRIOR 2
Standing with leg straight and foot facing the side- other leg placed in the front slightly bent - reach arms out to the side and then lift front arm up and arch body back

WARRIOR 3
Standing on one leg the other extended to the back – arms extended in front

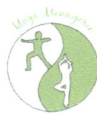

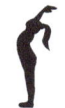

WATERFALL
Reach hands up and look up then roll down to bend in half

WHALE
Lying on the floor on your stomach - bend legs and bring feet up then turn the feet out to create a tail

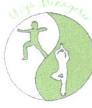

ADVENTURES IN KIDS YOGA

Flashcards

CUT OUT AND USE THESE FLASHCARDS AS ANOTHER FUN WAY TO LEARN POSES!

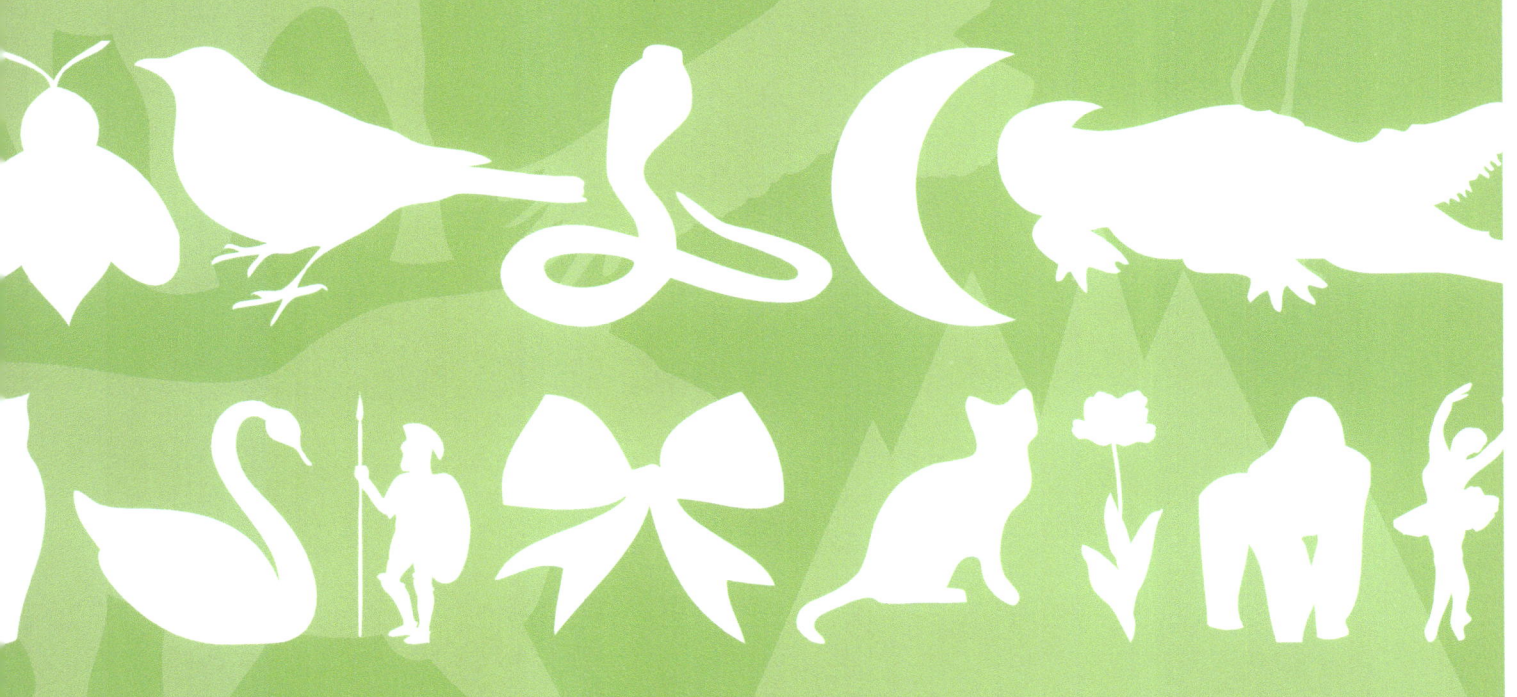

Flashcards

In this chapter, you will find flashcards on each page. The layout is set up so that when you cut the flashcard out for personal use, the front image will correspond with the image on the back. It's all set up for you to cut out end enjoy!

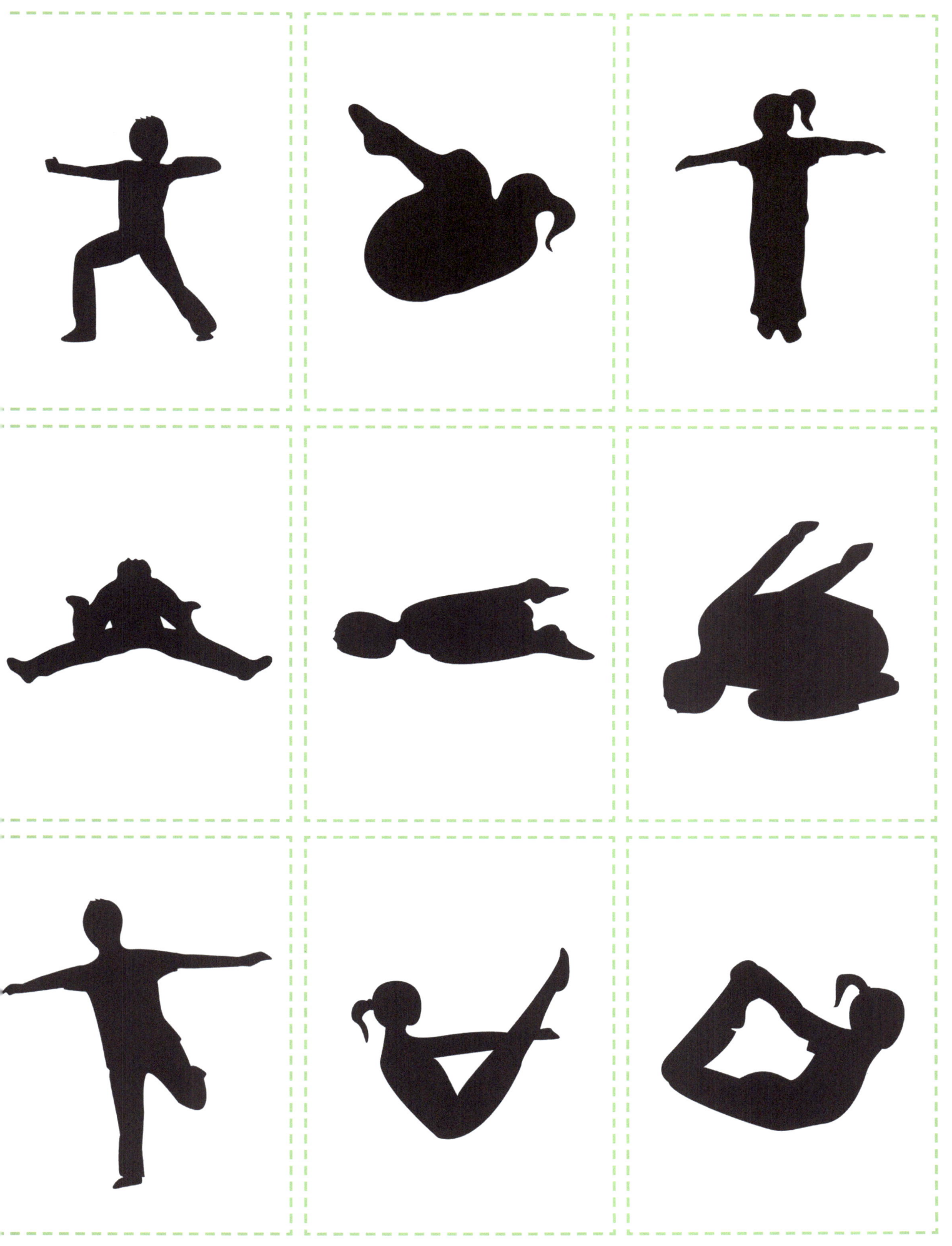

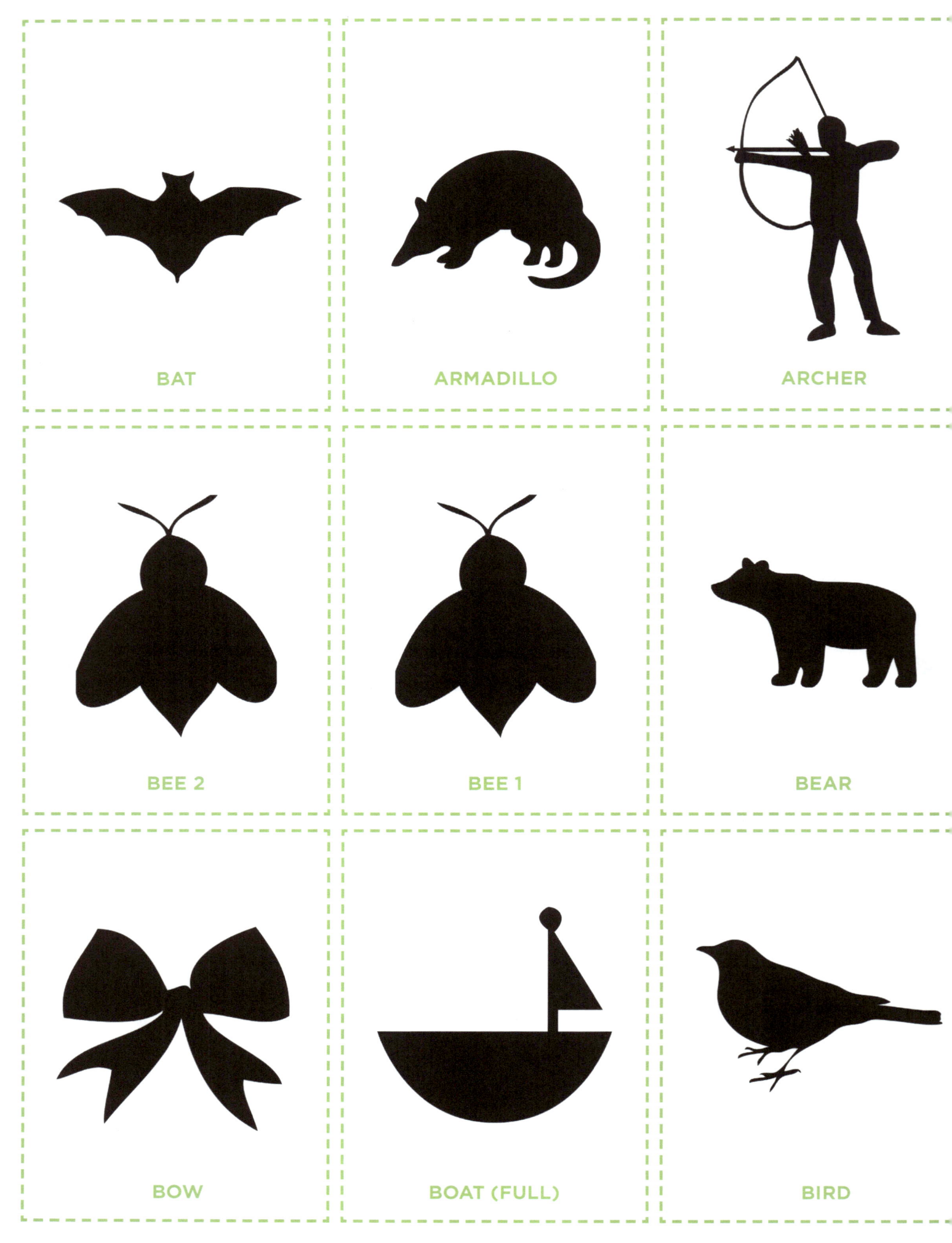

BAT

ARMADILLO

ARCHER

BEE 2

BEE 1

BEAR

BOW

BOAT (FULL)

BIRD

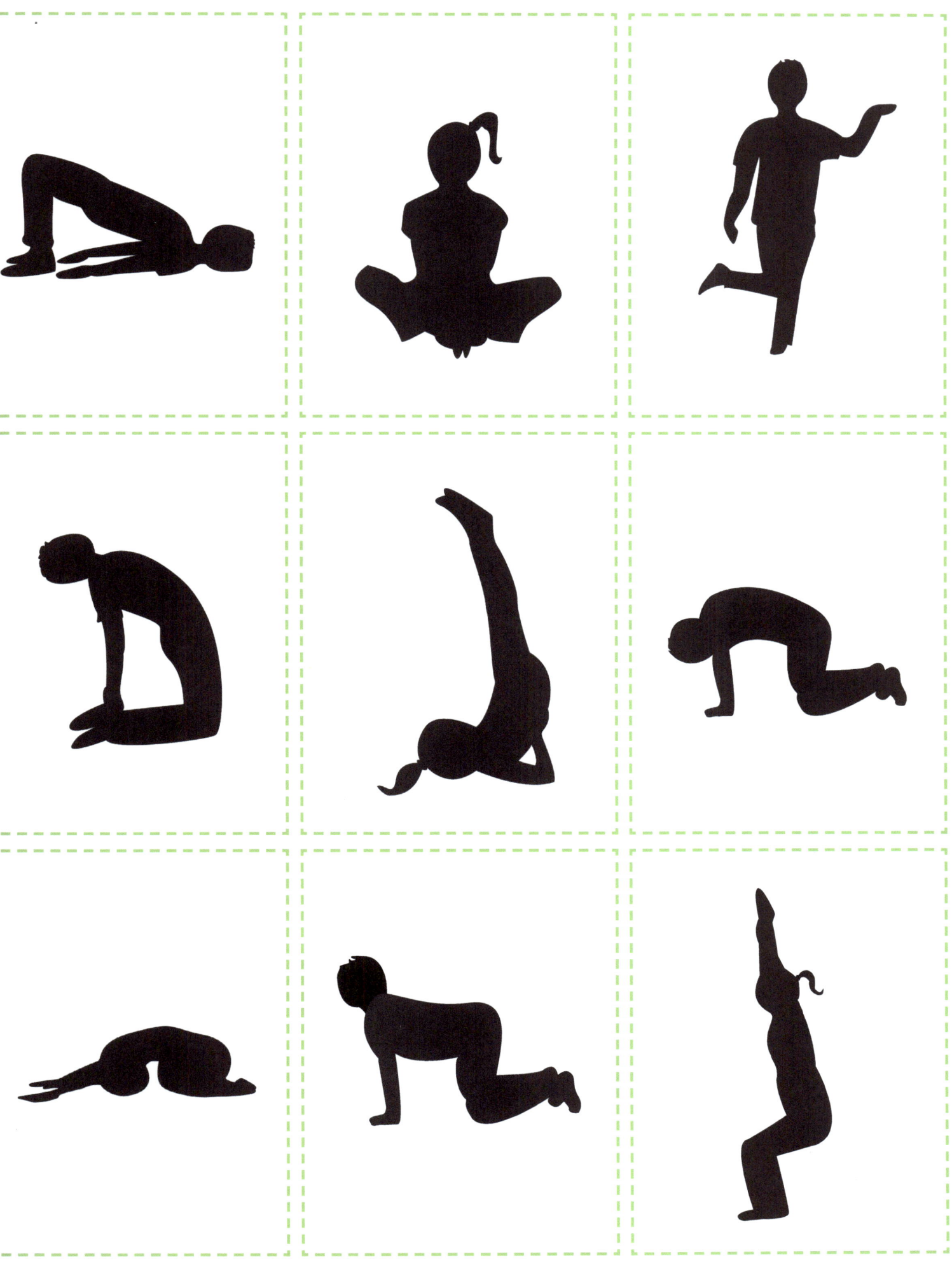

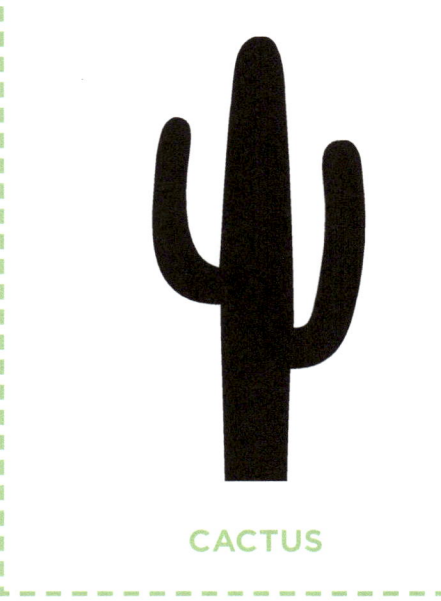

CACTUS

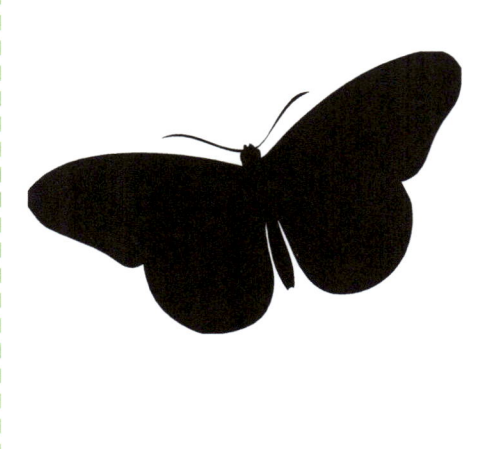

BUTTERFLY

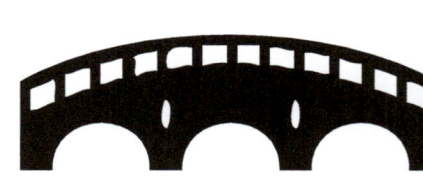

BRIDGE

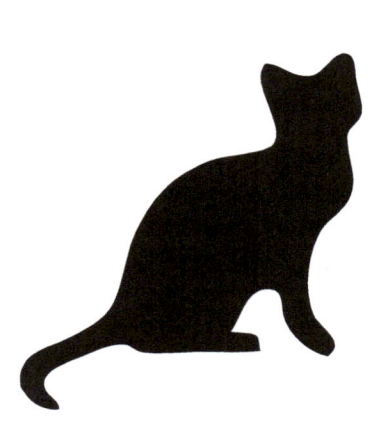
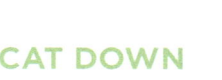

CAT DOWN

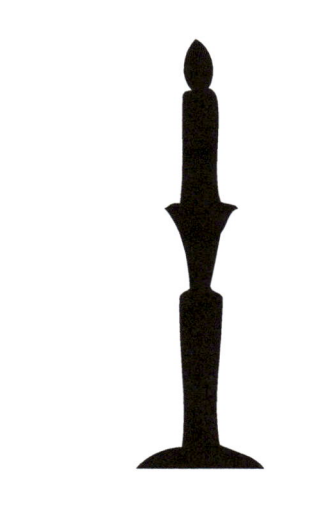

CANDLESTICK

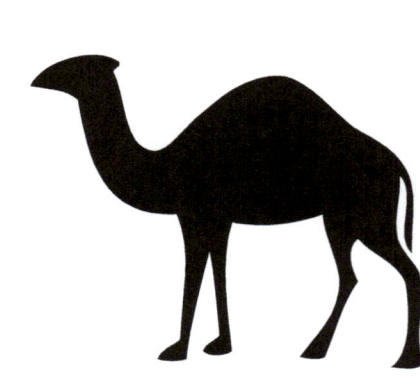

CAMEL

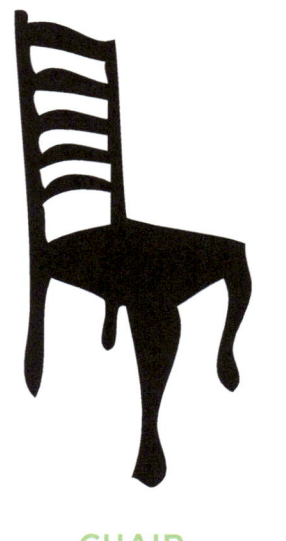

CHAIR

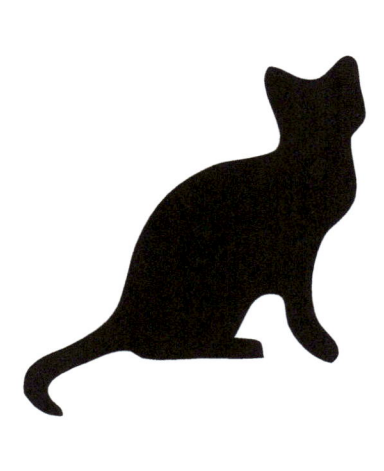

CAT UP

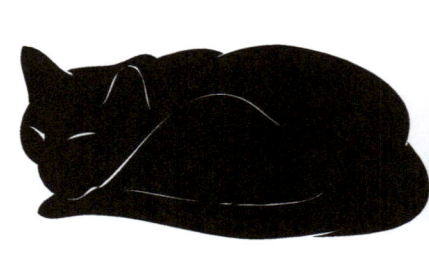

CAT SLEEPING

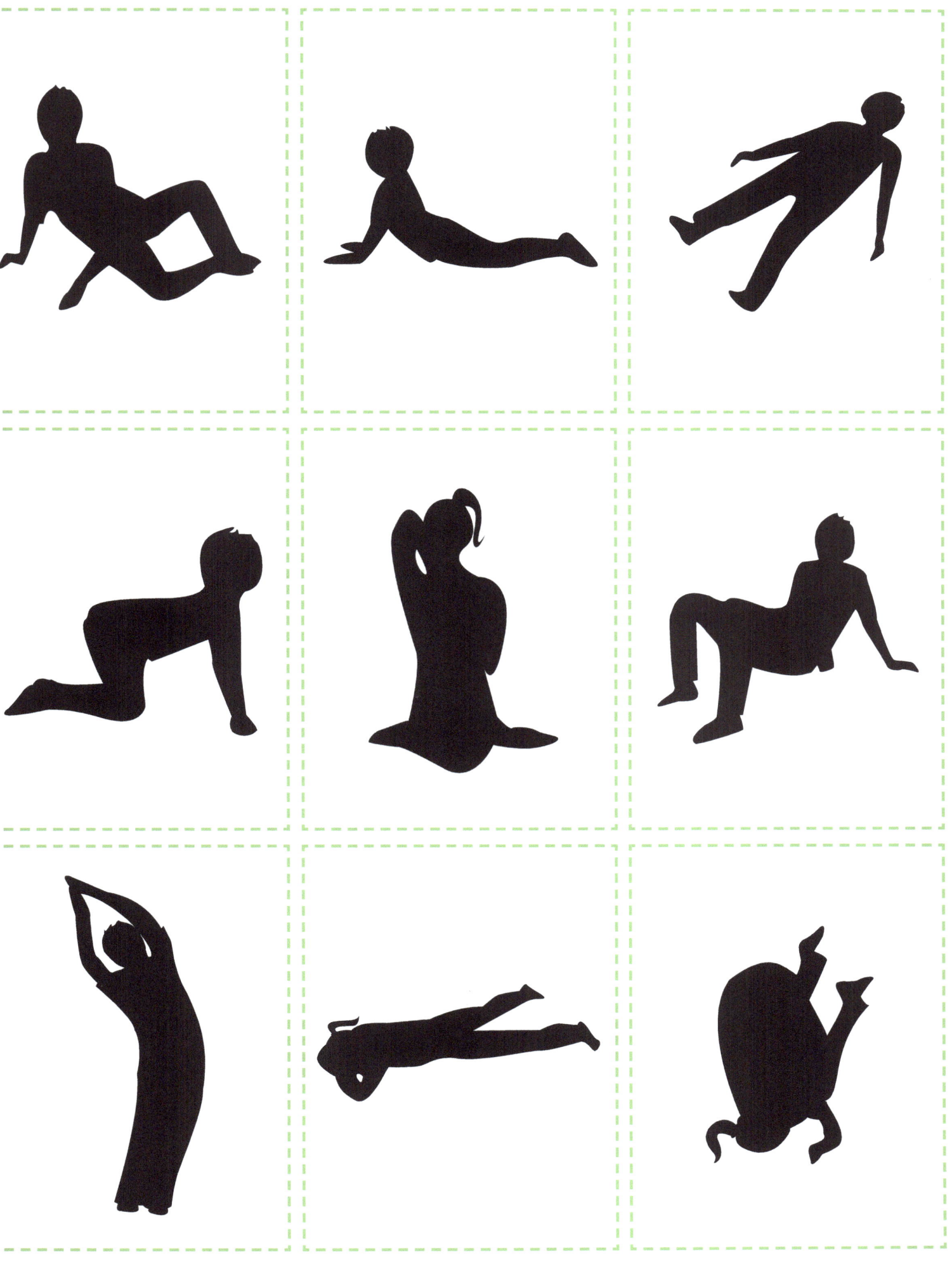

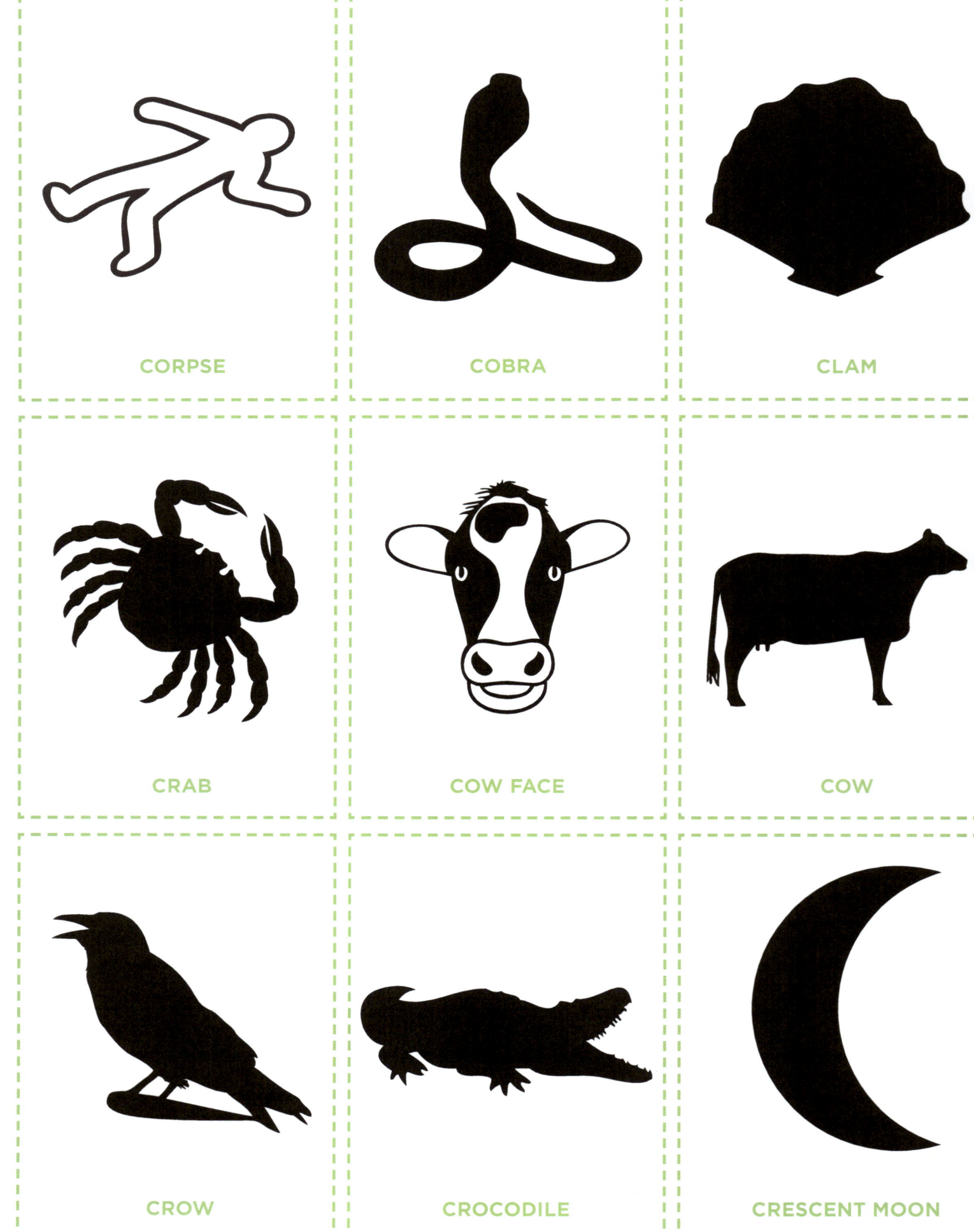

CORPSE

COBRA

CLAM

CRAB

COW FACE

COW

CROW

CROCODILE

CRESCENT MOON

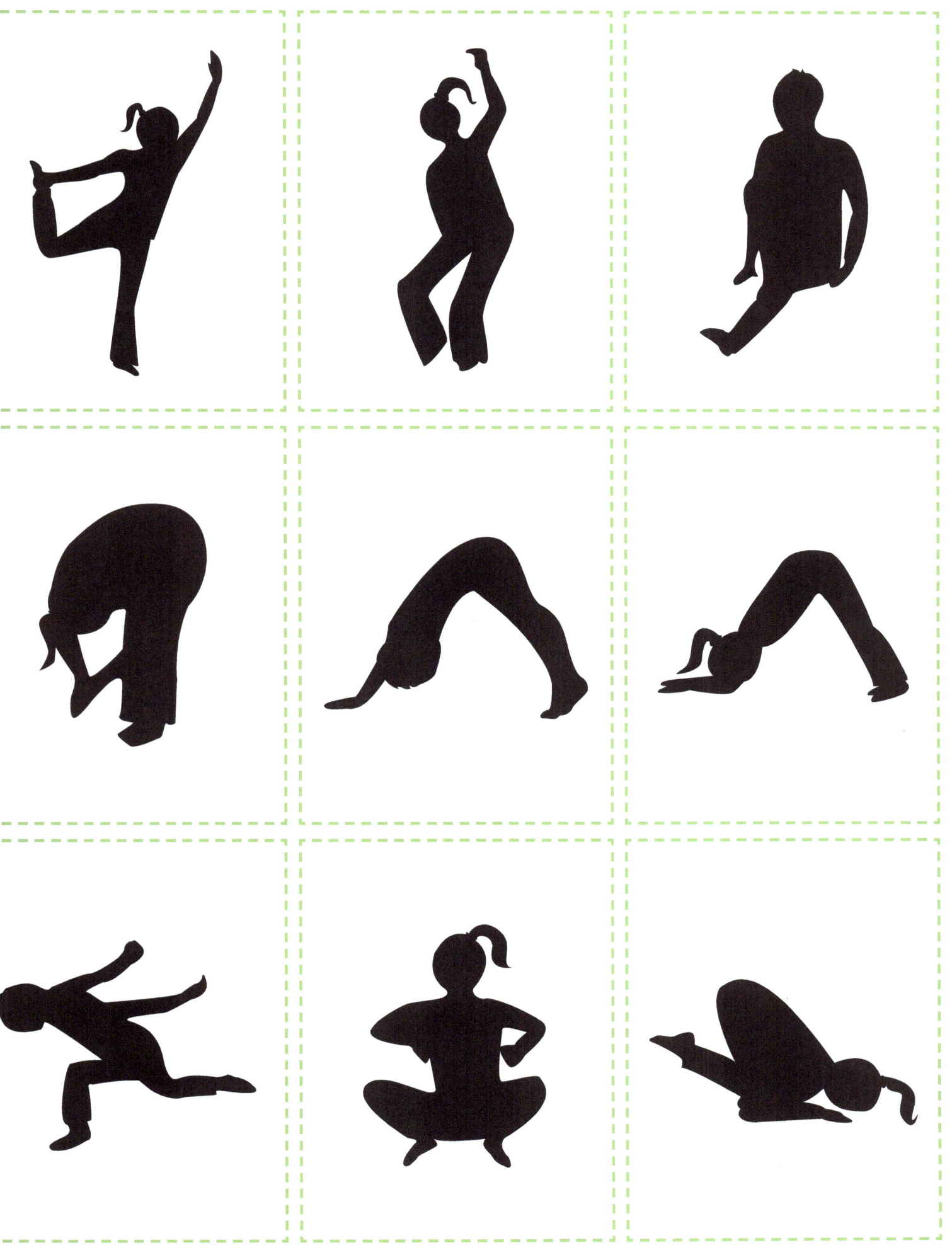

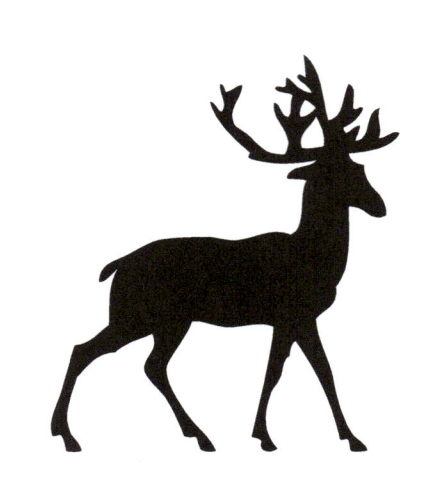

DEER

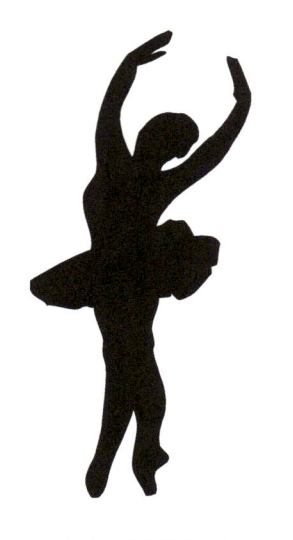

DANCER 2

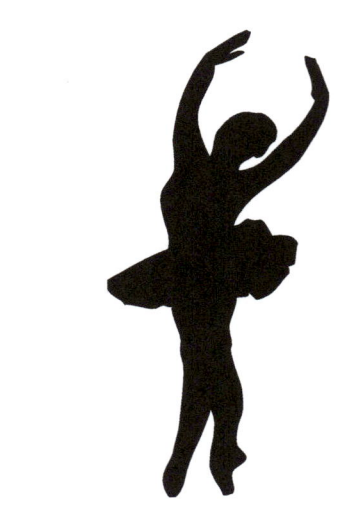

DANCER 1

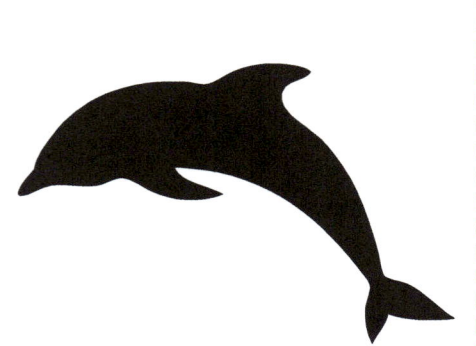

DOLPHIN

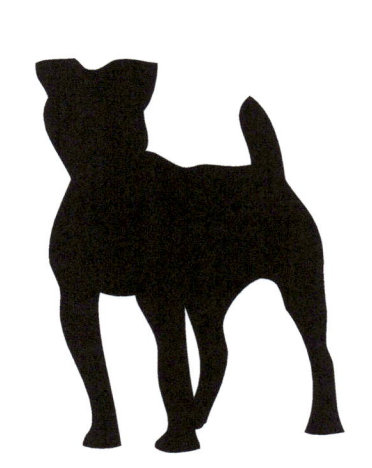

DOG

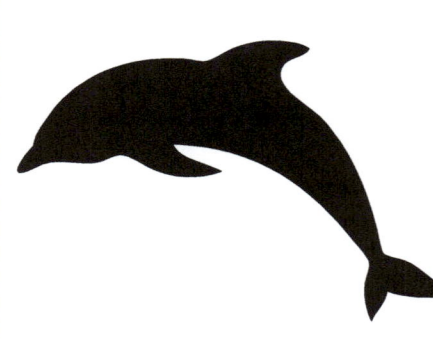

DIVING DOLPHIN

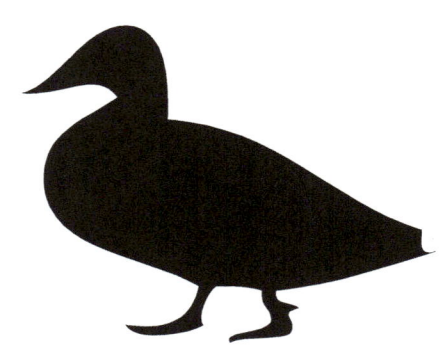

DUCK 2

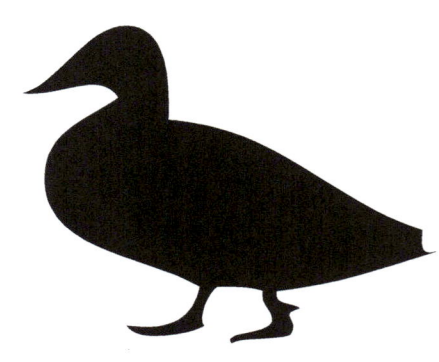

DUCK 1

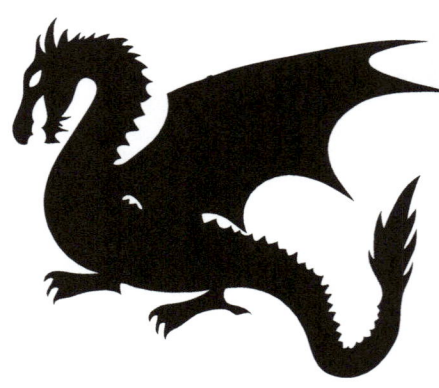

DRAGON

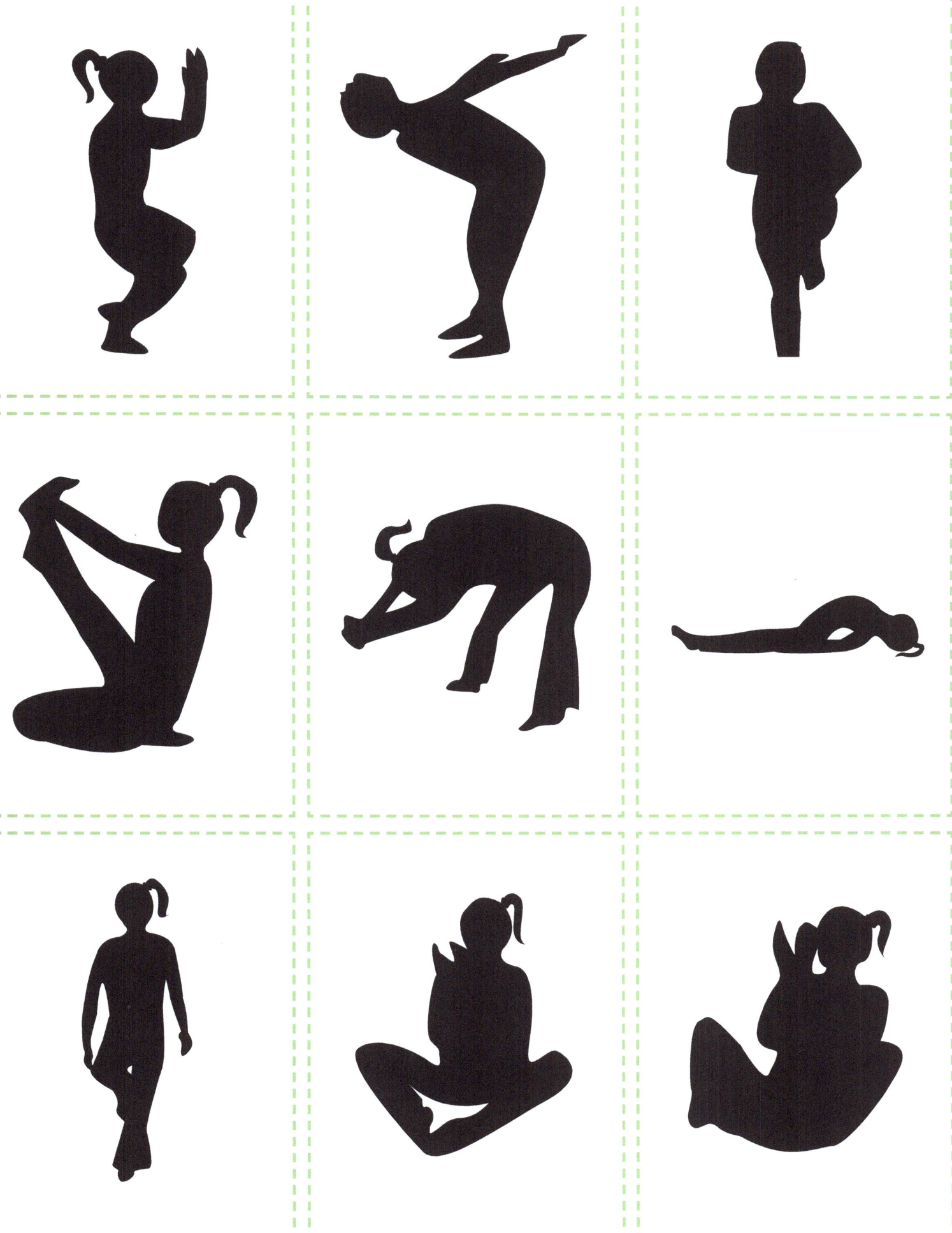

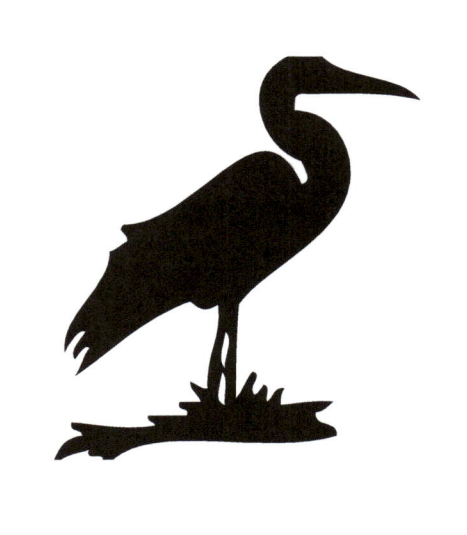

EGRET 1

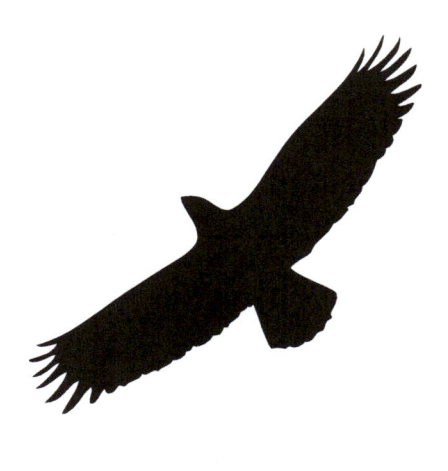

EAGLE 2

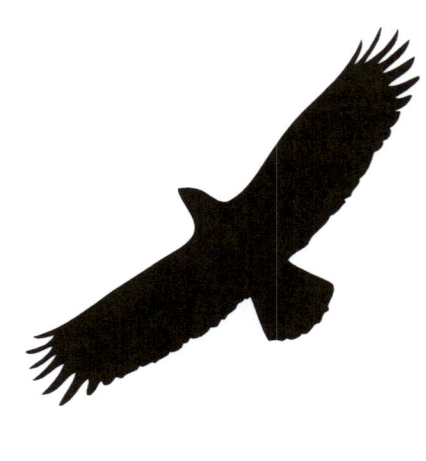

EAGLE 1

FISH

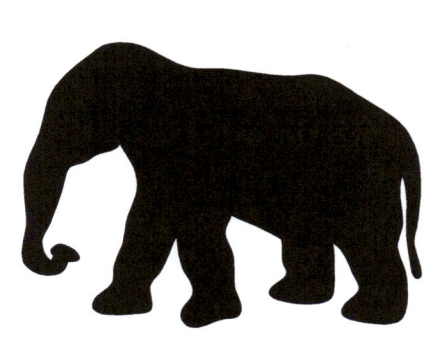

ELEPHANT

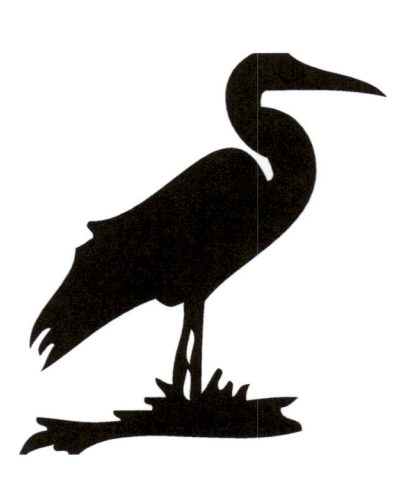

EGRET 2

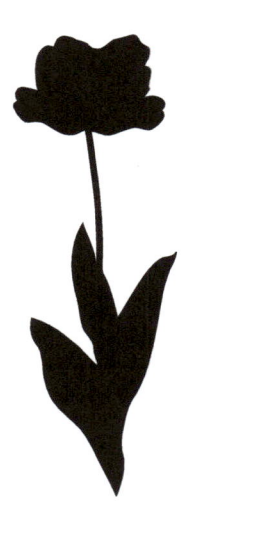

FLOWER 2

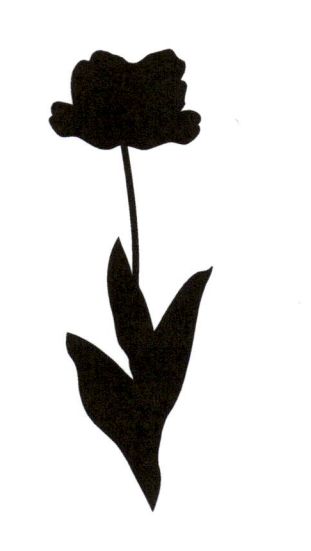

FLOWER 1

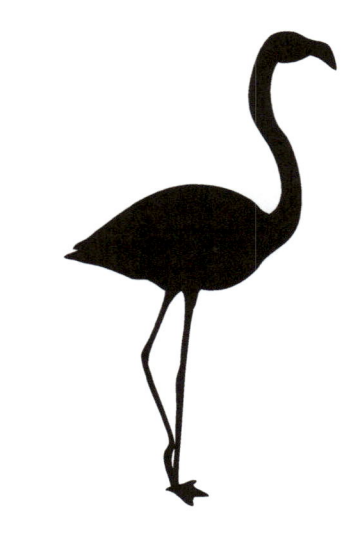

FLAMINGO

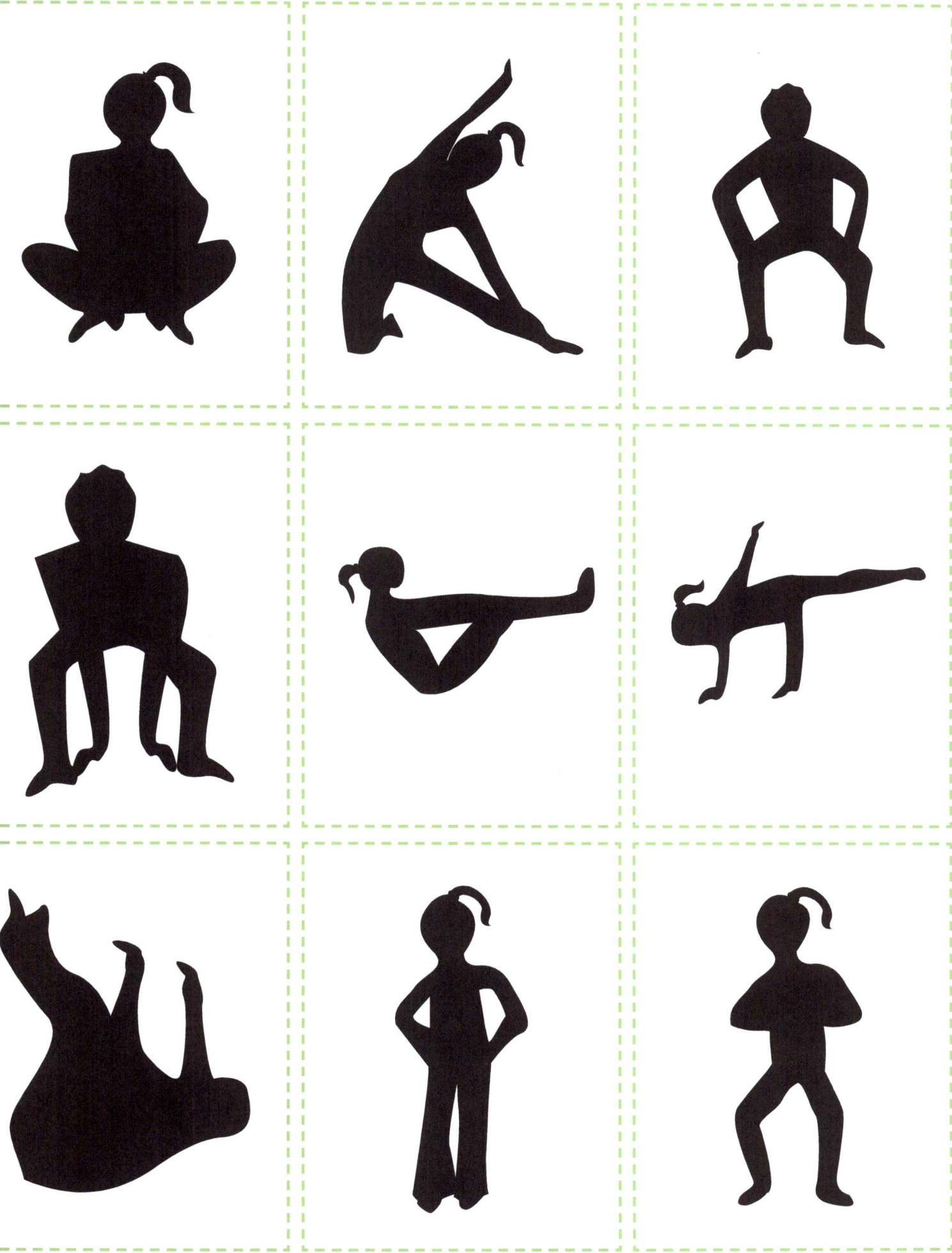

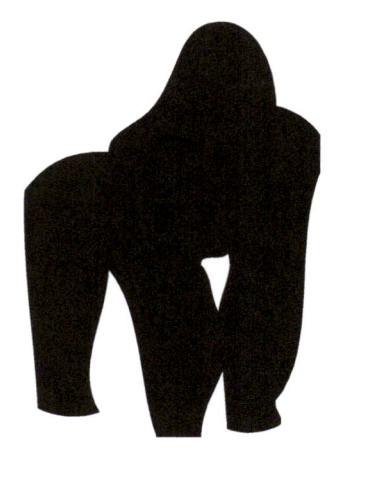

GORILLA 1

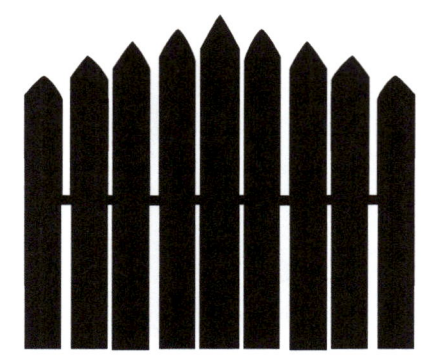

GATELATCH

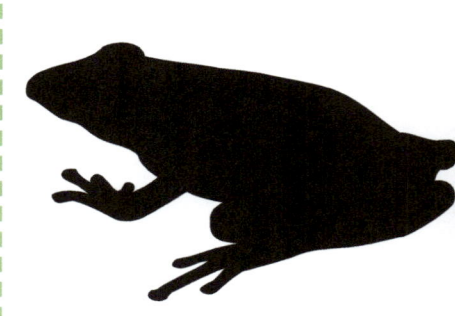

FROG

HALF MOON

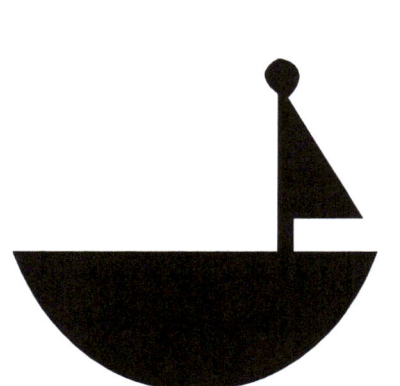

HALF BOAT

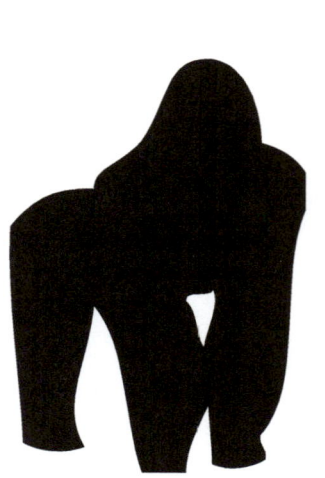

GORILLA 2

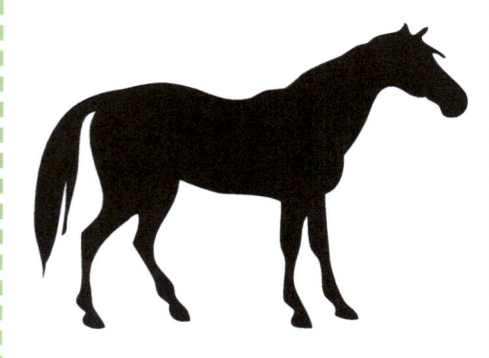

HORSE

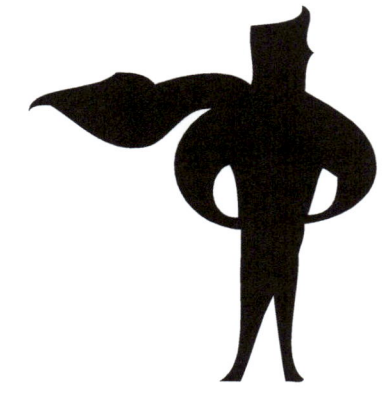

HERO

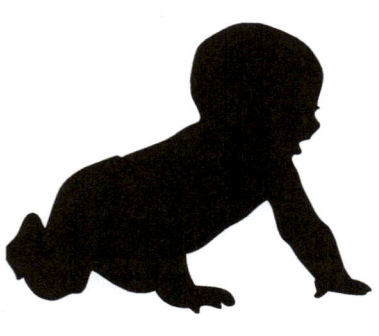

HAPPY BABY

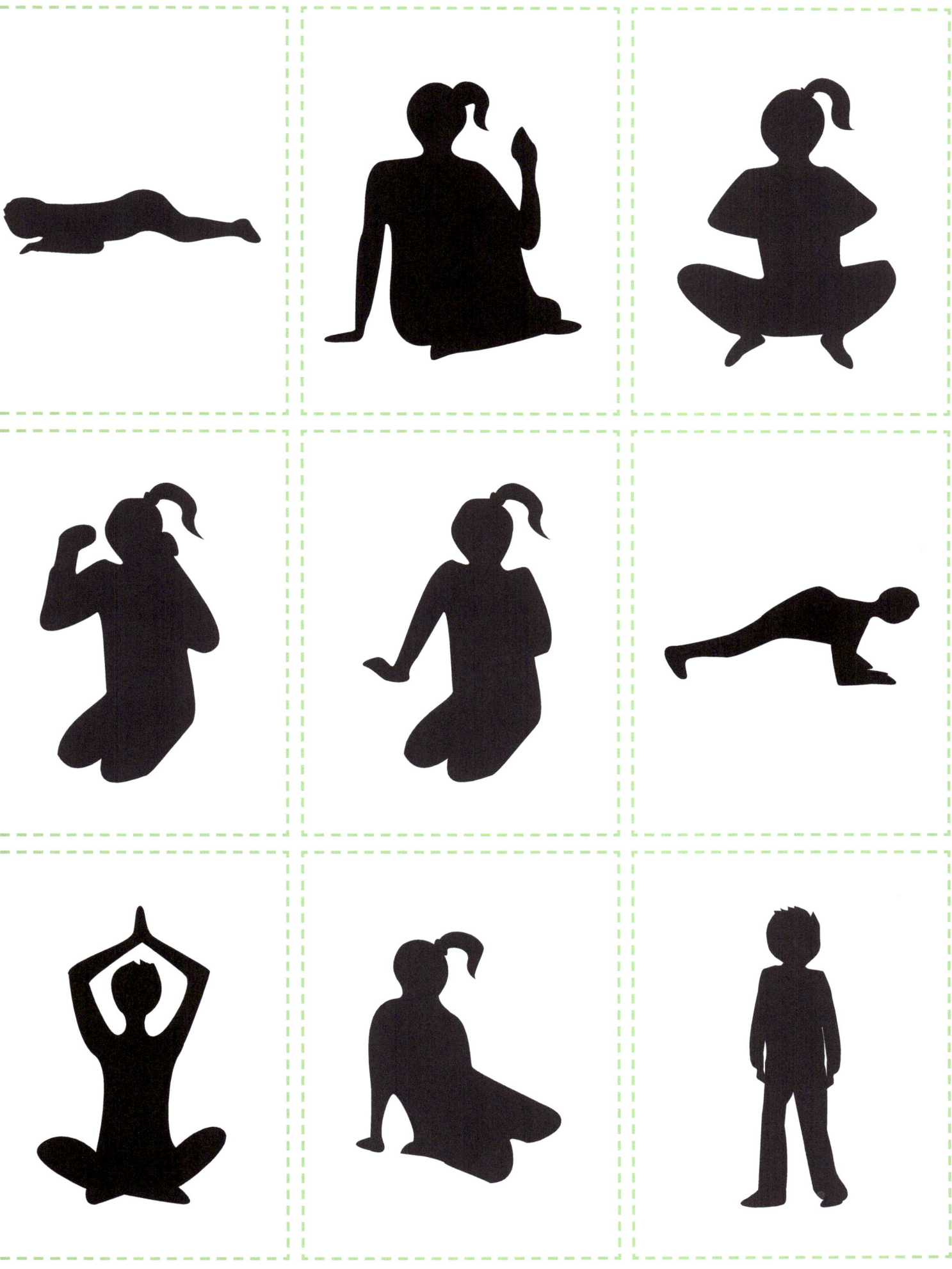

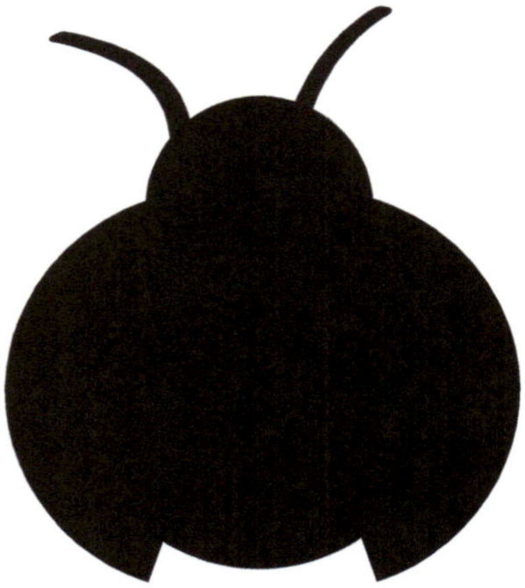

LADYBUG

KING OF FISH

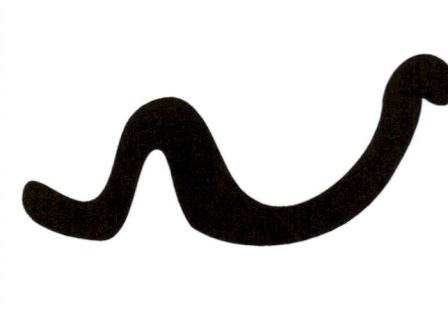

INCHWORM

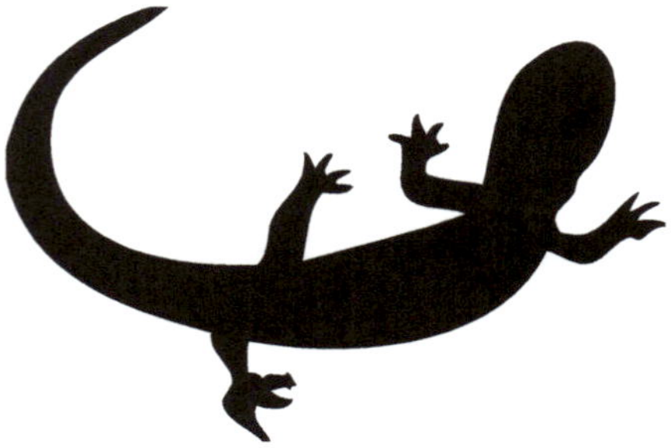

LIZARD

LION 2

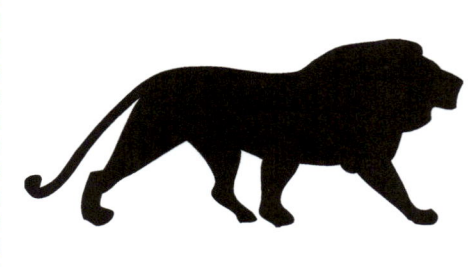

LION 1

MOUNTAIN

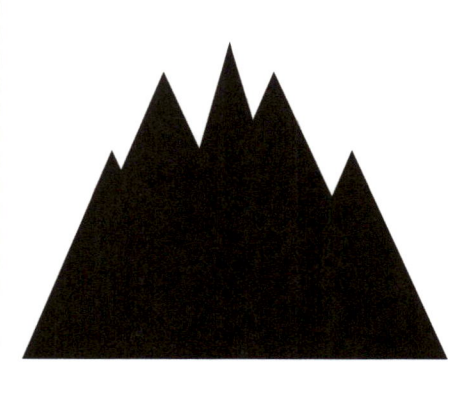

MERMAID

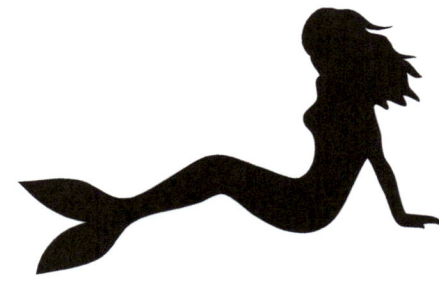

LOTUS

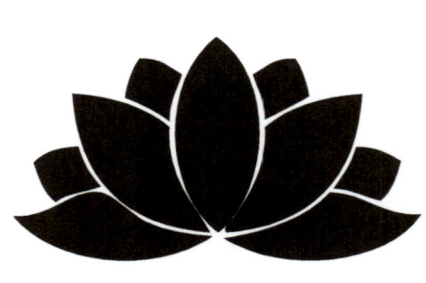

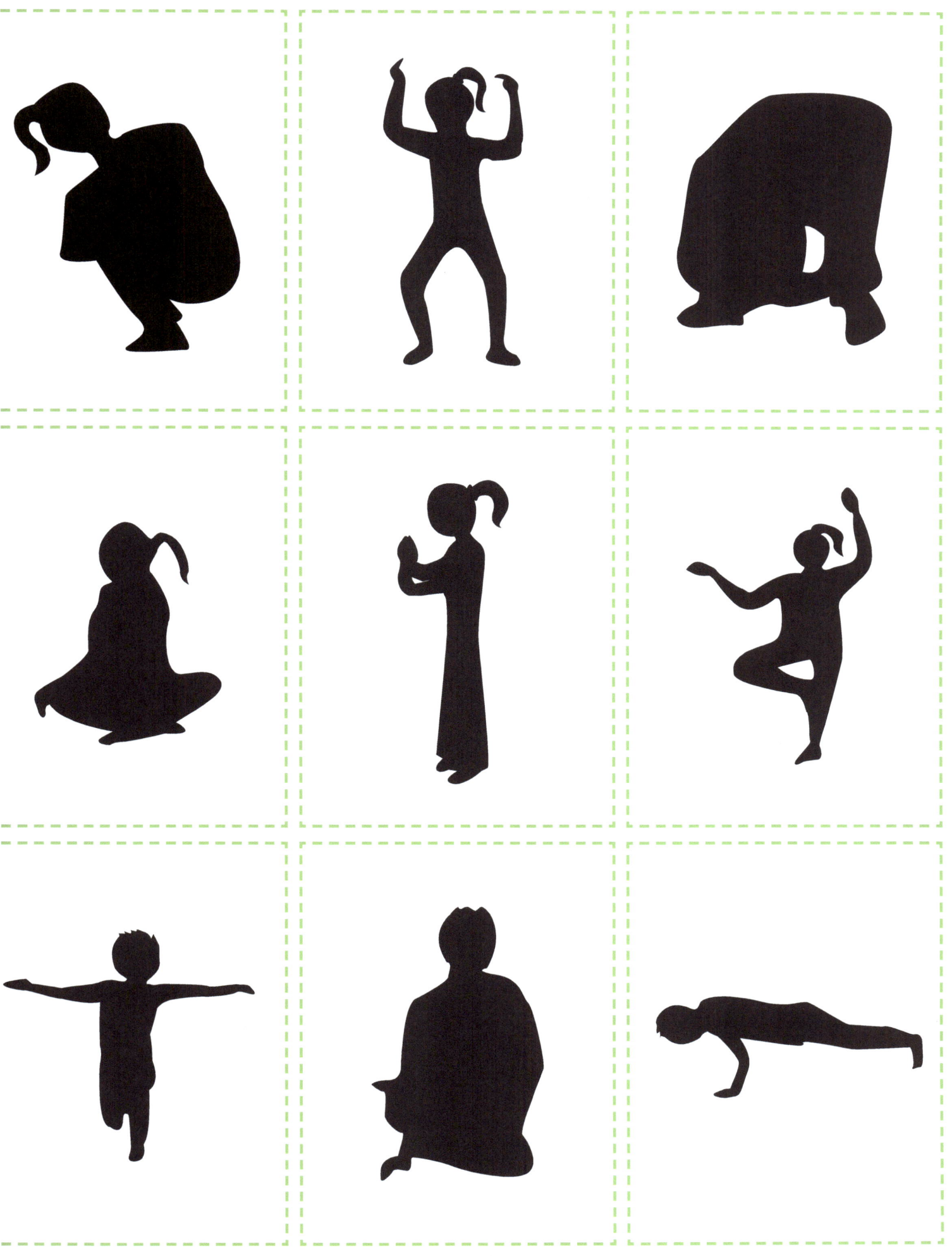

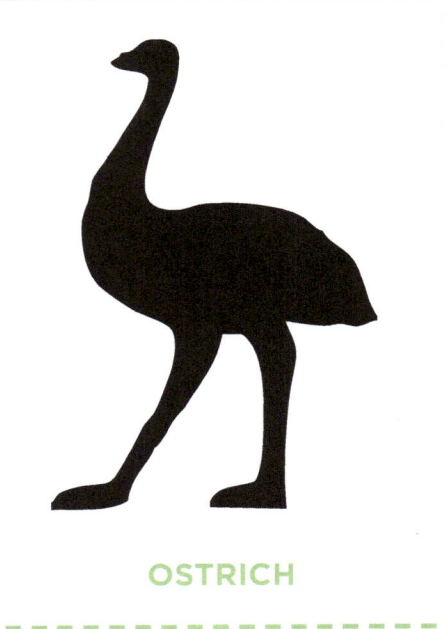

OSTRICH

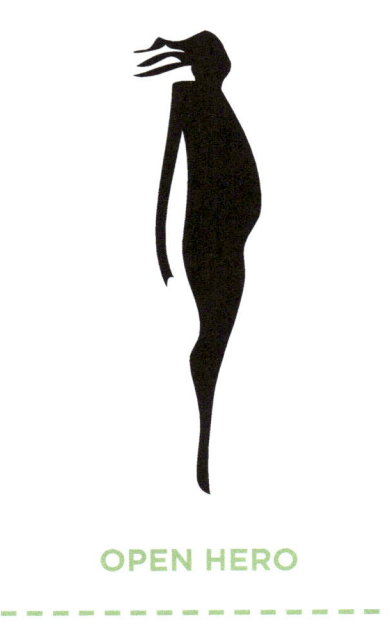

OPEN HERO

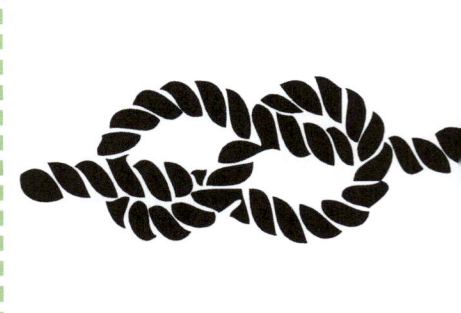

NOOSE

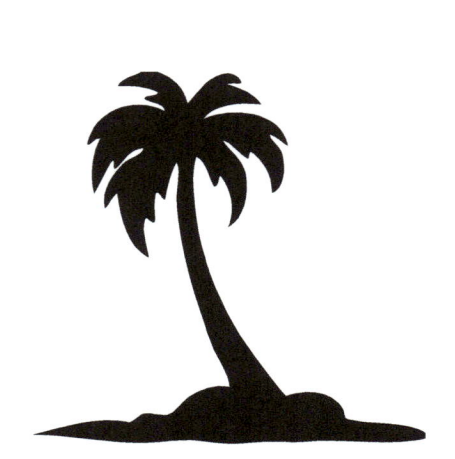
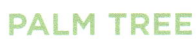

PALM TREE

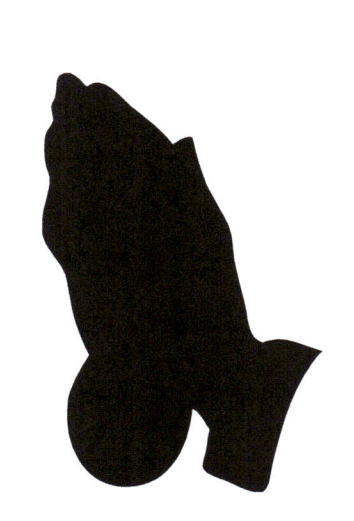

PALM PRESS

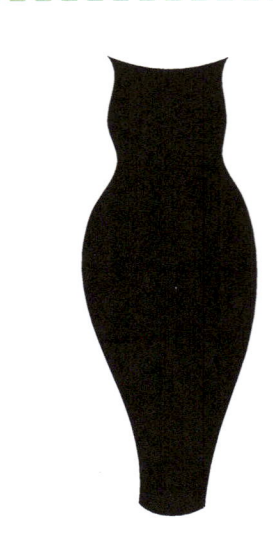

OWL

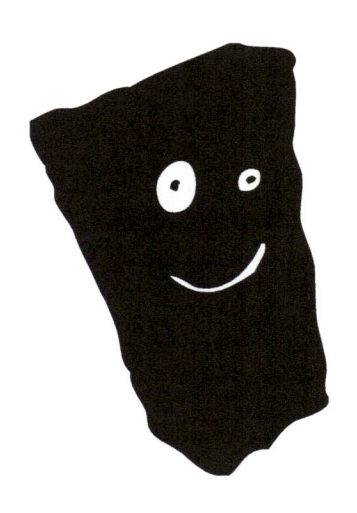

PLANK

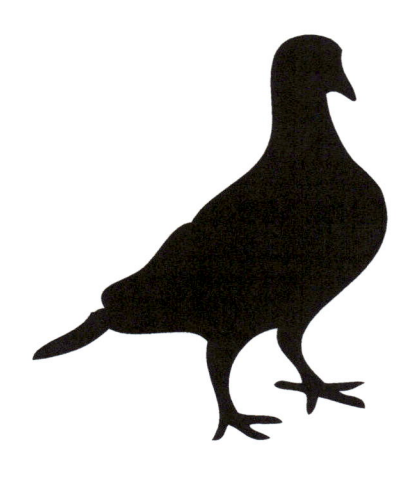

PIGEON

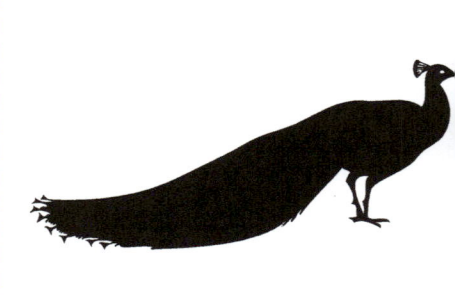

PEACOCK

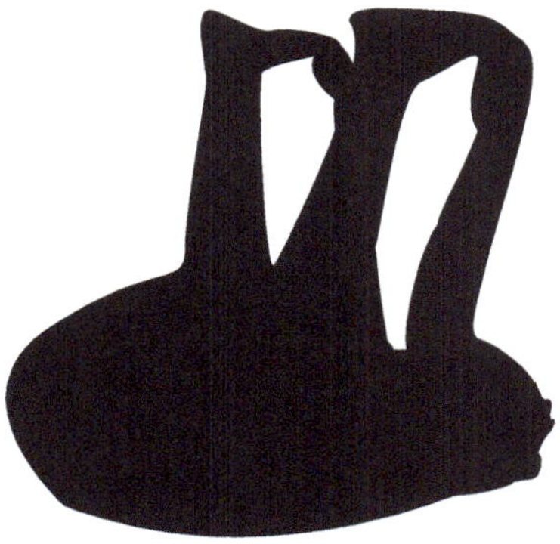

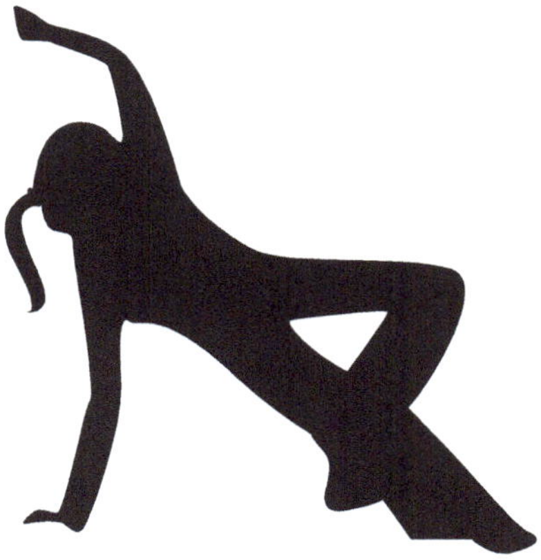

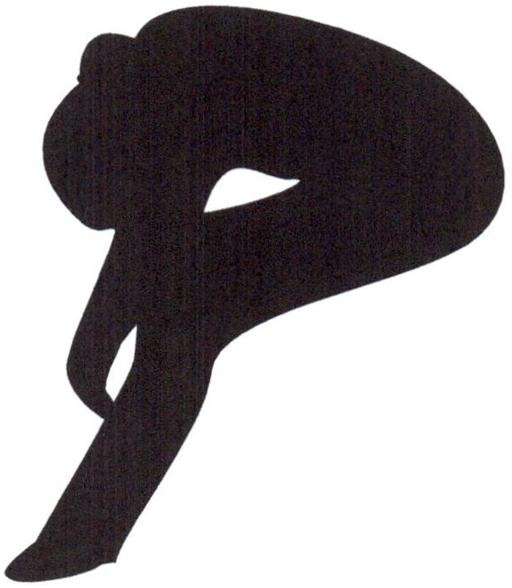

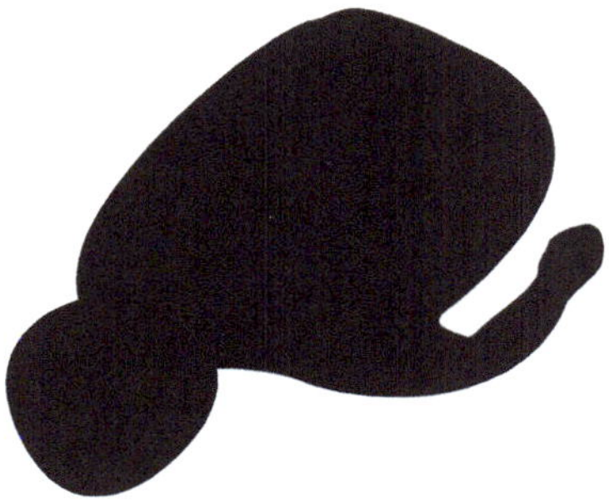

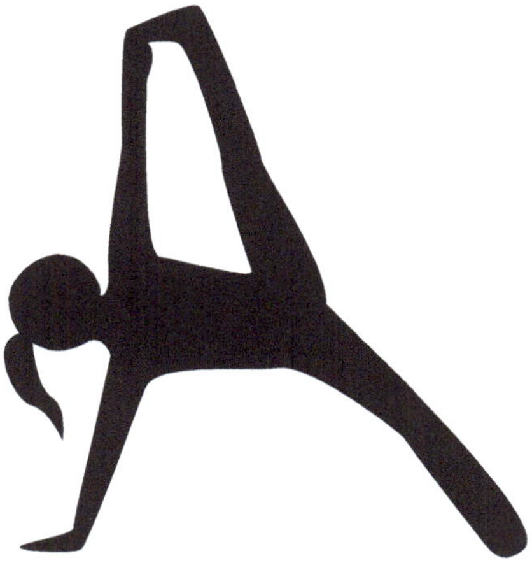

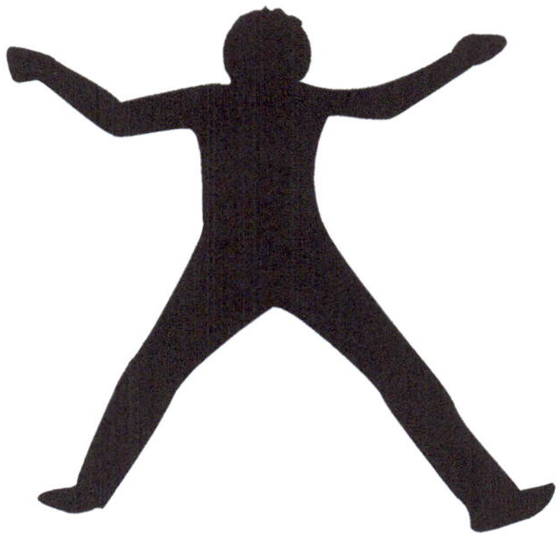

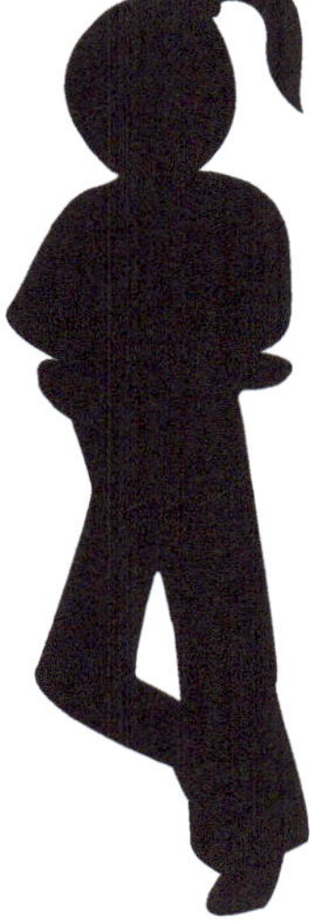

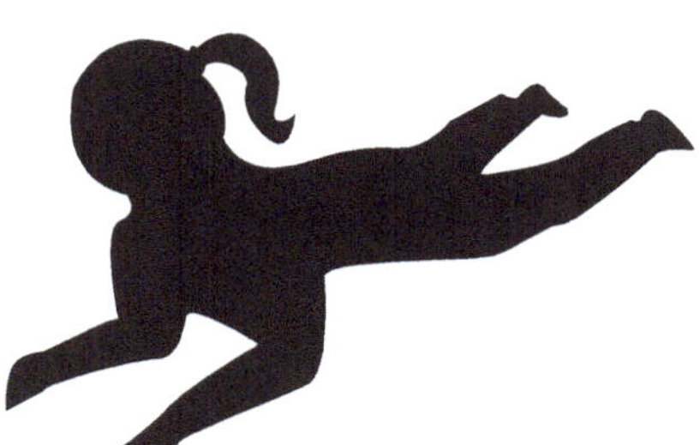

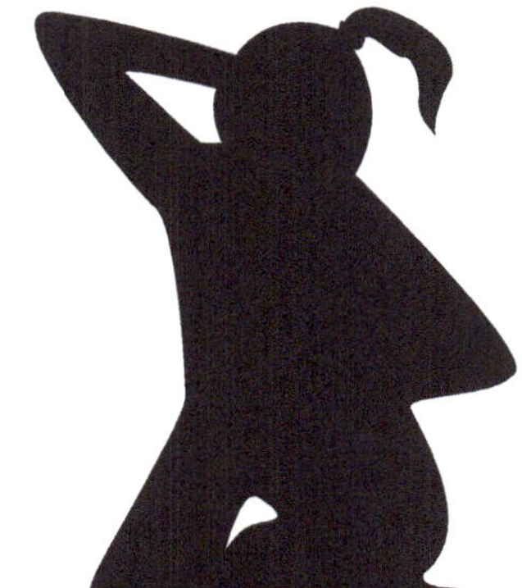

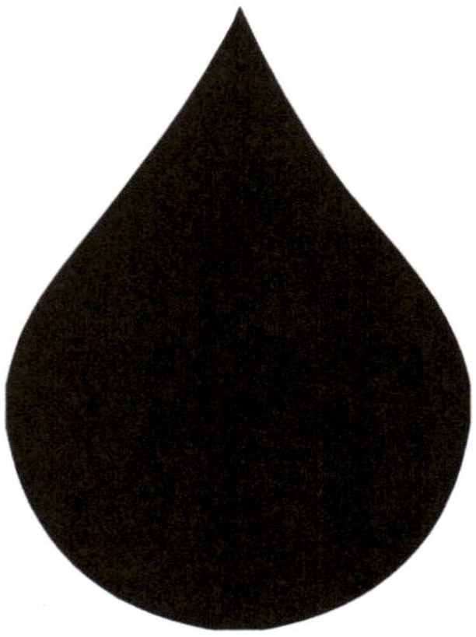

RAINDROP

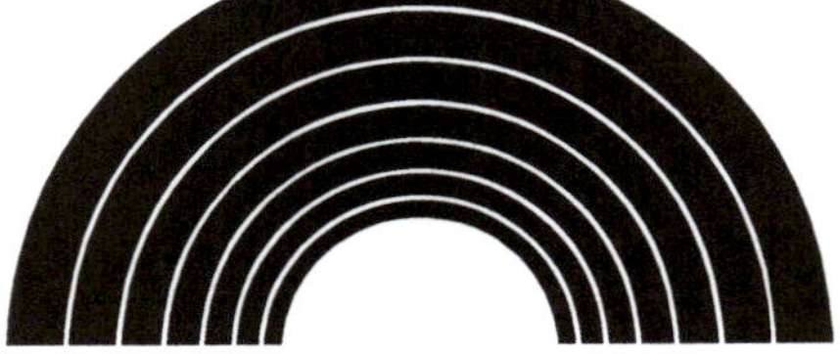

RAINBOW

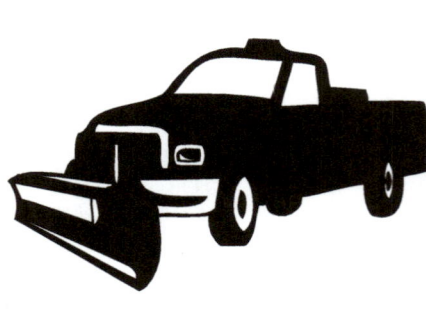

PLOW

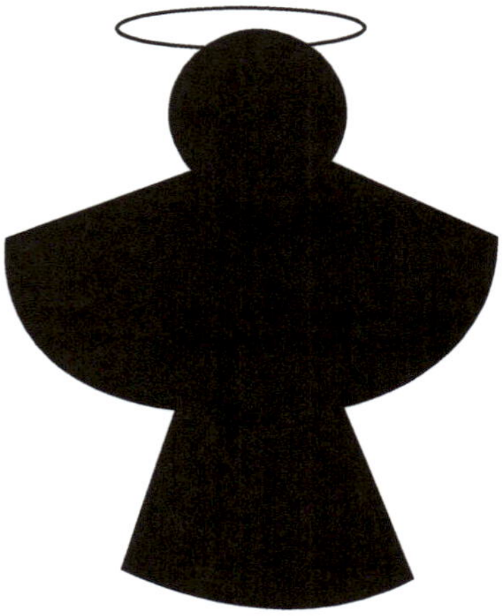

SAND ANGEL

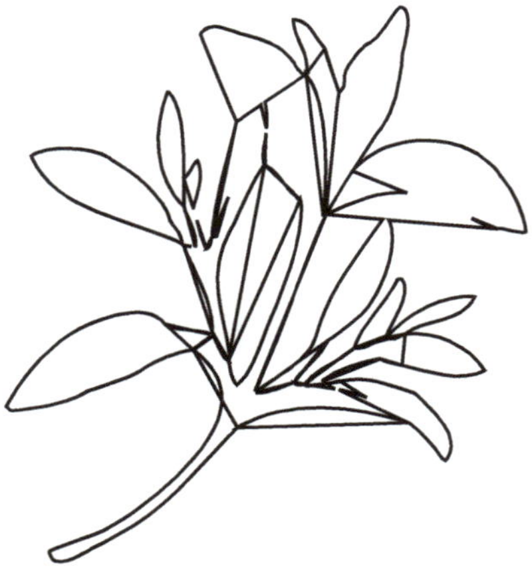

SAGE

ROCK

SEASHELL

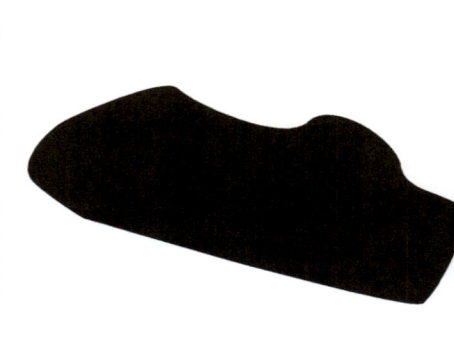

SEAL

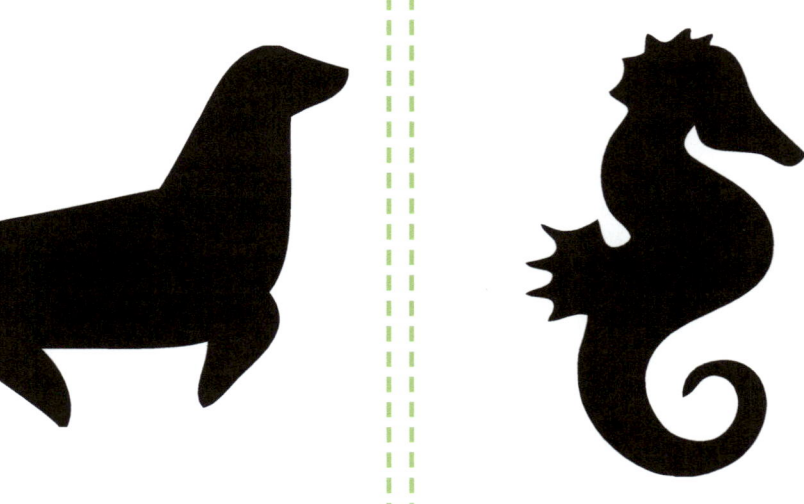

SEAHORSE

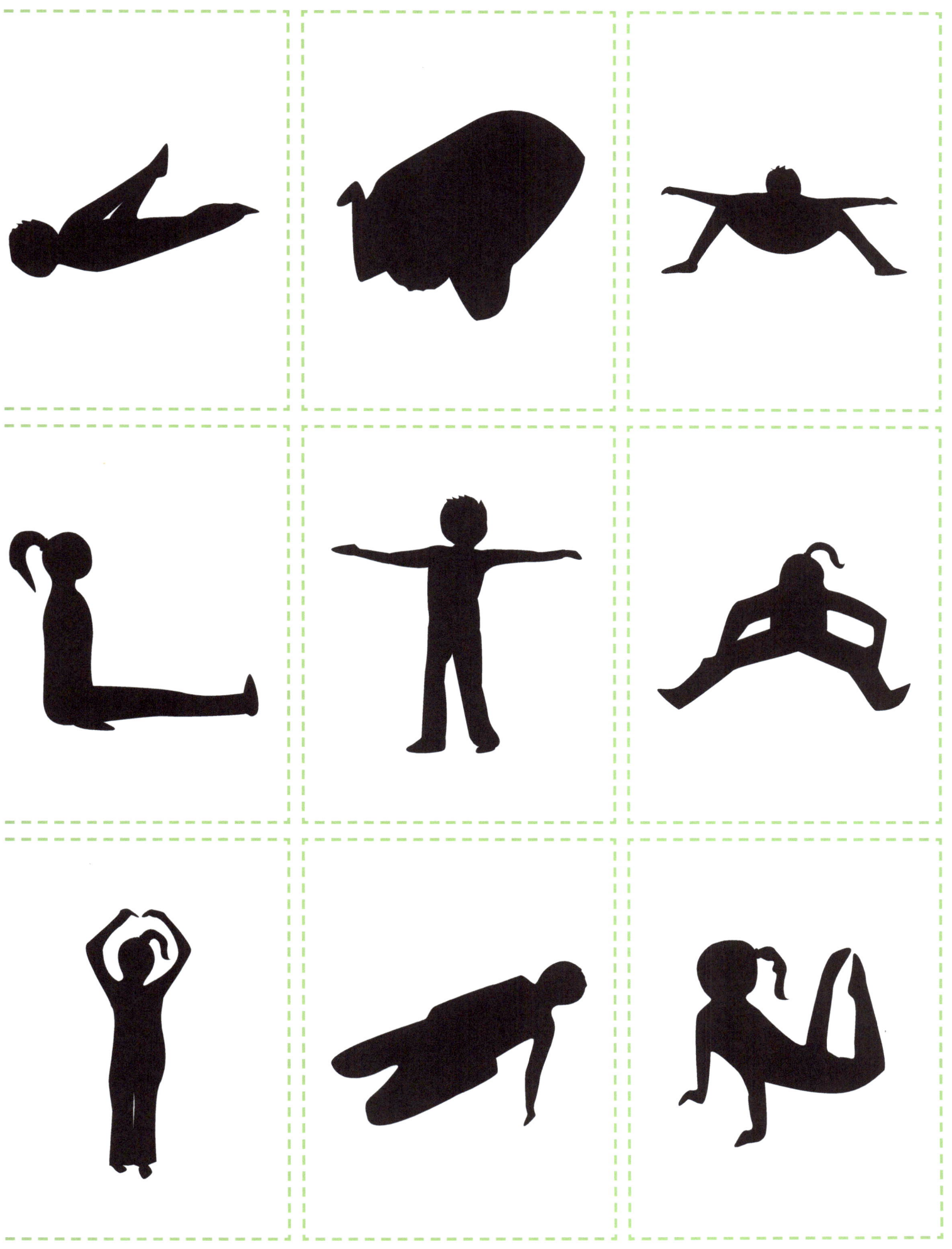

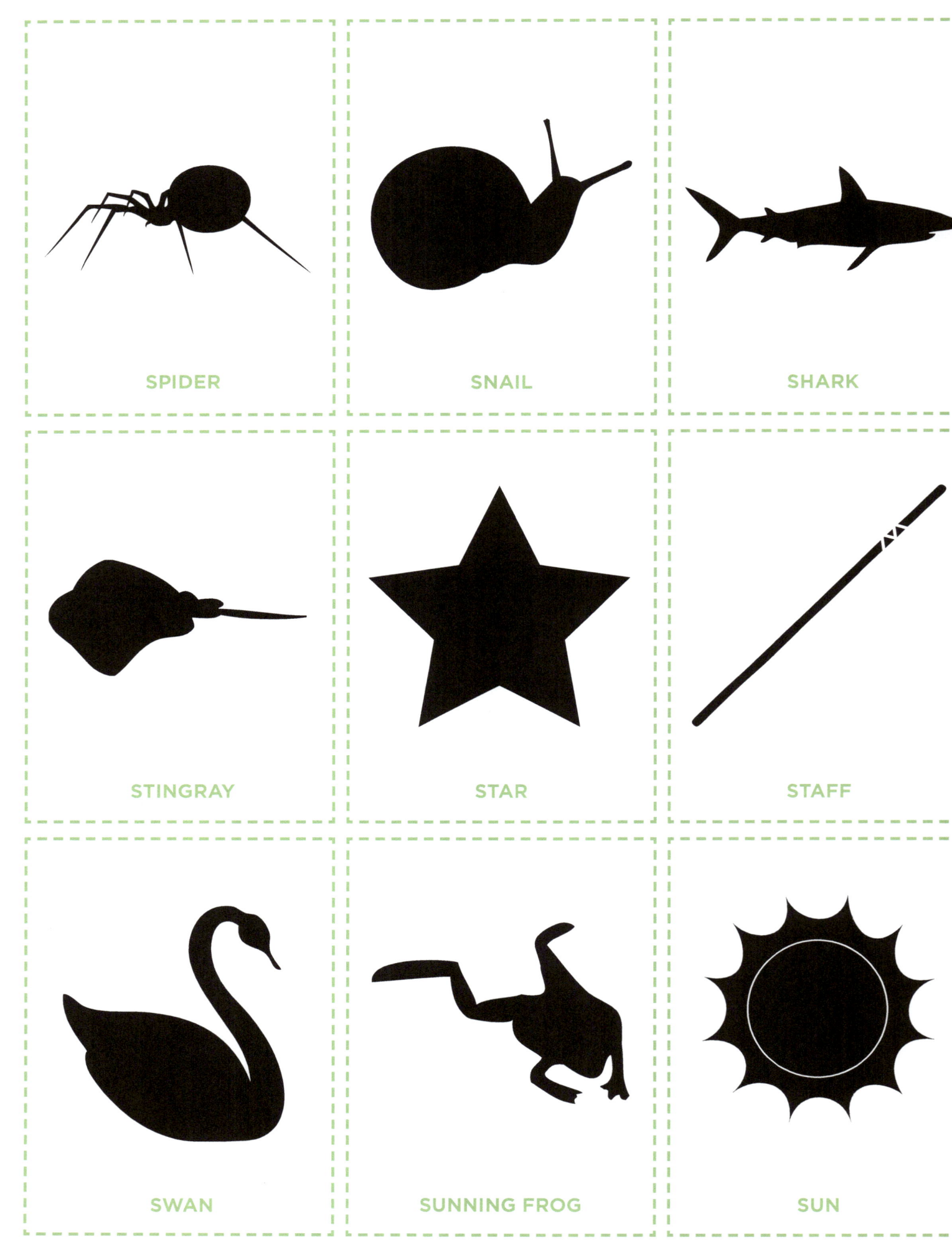

SPIDER

SNAIL

SHARK

STINGRAY

STAR

STAFF

SWAN

SUNNING FROG

SUN

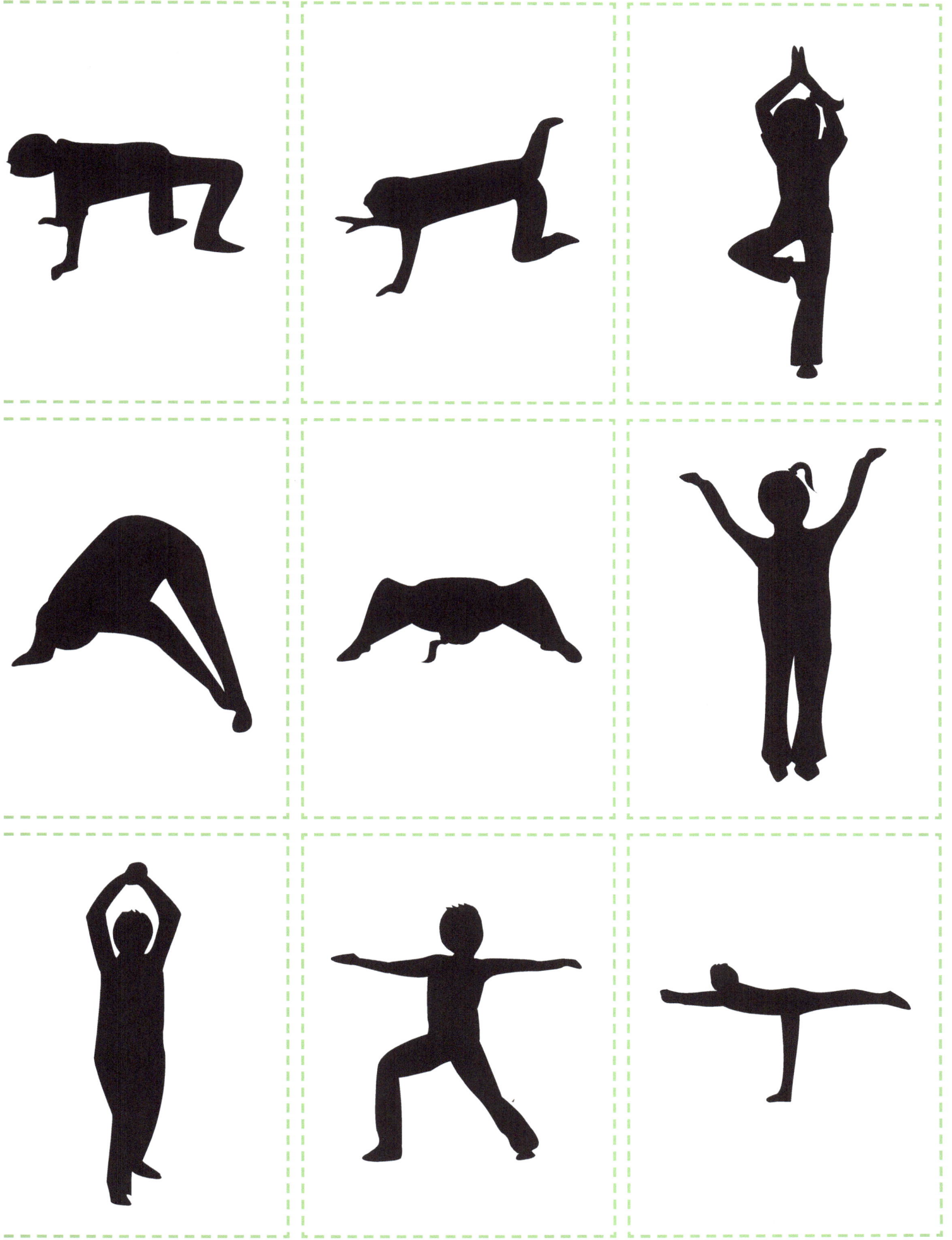

TREE

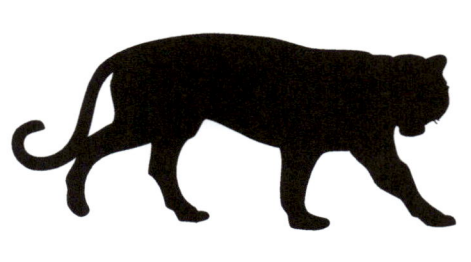

TIGER

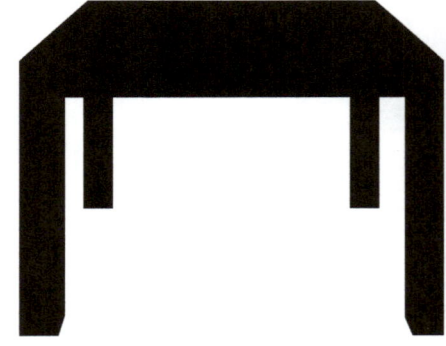

TABLE

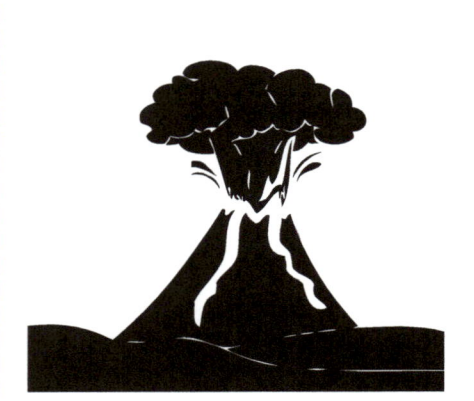

VOLCANO

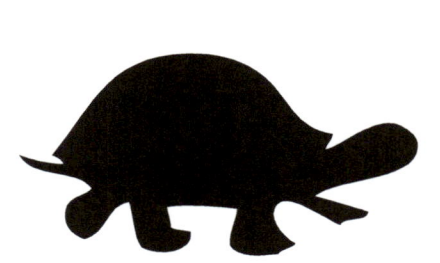

TURTLE

TRIANGLE

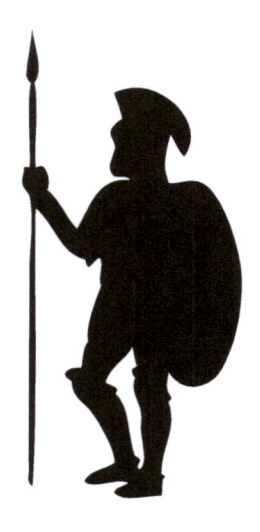

WARRIOR 3

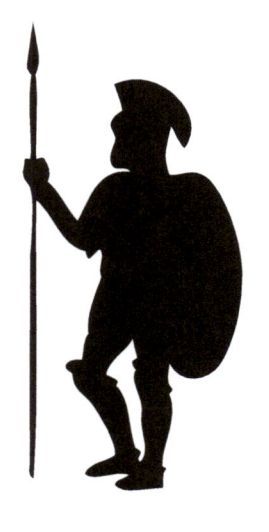

WARRIOR 2

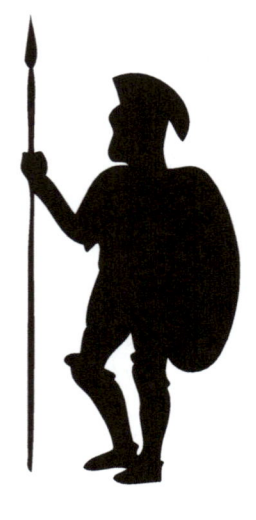

WARRIOR 1

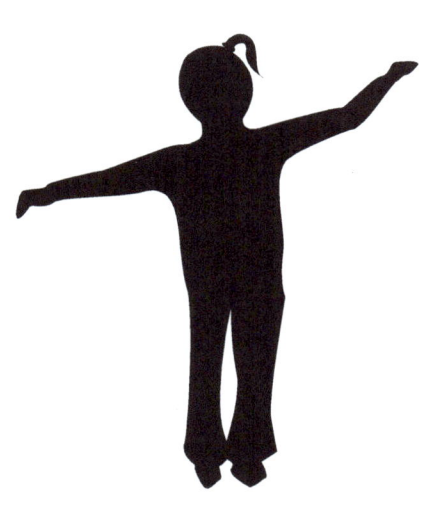

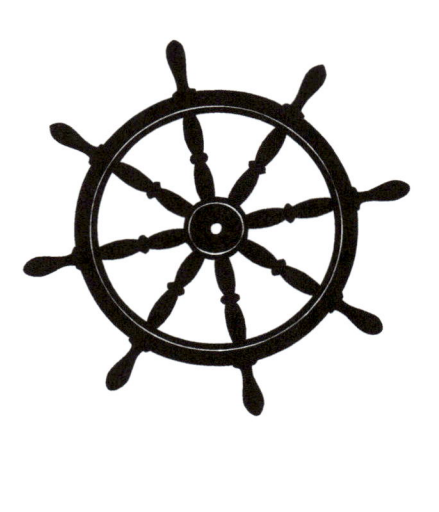

WHEEL

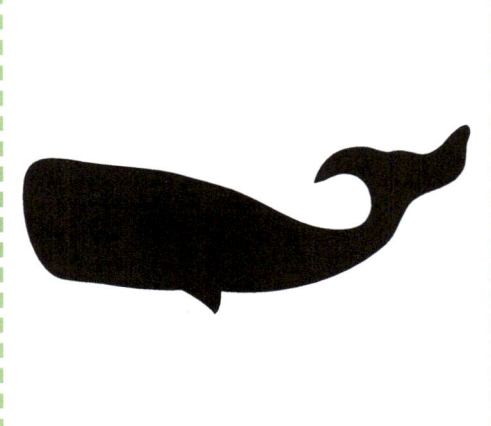
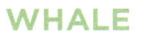

WHALE

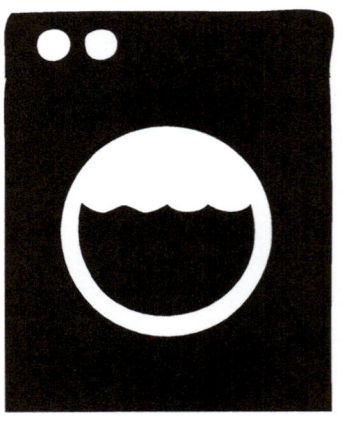

WASHING MACHINE

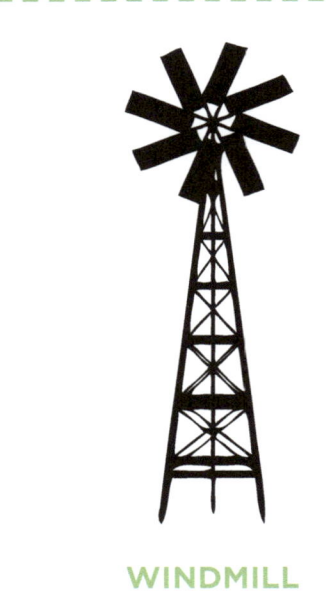

WINDMILL

About the Author

Con reprehe ndellore exerspi enimolupta sanimo dolorerate accum diti unt rehenet erro mos et explitisque se erit lique rest repro digenderum vercimus ea volupta tinctiam quis ereptus molum invererrupta nus aliscii scidita diosseque quis idunti asitia volupta tibus, nusam lab in porepel estibus.

Eriae maio. Occabor ad magnihi lloritae pa voluptis aut quia doluptae se nus vent verrovidel illessi molentiuntem vel in reped mostis si re eium quid unt ea voluptae lati asinvelendit vent lab il maios eume nobit quiatiur, volori omnis evenditas doluptur, que eos eumquatem fugit lant unt vella sincto eum, voluptatur, que eici restota speribus voloribus vitatem laboraeste et aliquam eius magnat il magnime et modit asperias sa dolorrum estia nonsedi utem non nist eum quam quam quuntius, ute sed qui torro temquat quamus.

Ecab il in necae reptur, quos quis dolenis aut fugit fugitent lit es molorestium nobit et est vernat hil int.

Quid magnate mporepu daectem quatibus delia il ium, con recum, consequist, que doluptiates voluptatate elique qui dis ilibus dolor aut veliqui aut etusciis debit quam core provid enimagnam fugiatis preprepre plicae niminul litios aut quam, audandi scipist, quos aliam erum restium senis et, si dolorio idio tet, officil magnima gnimet harchit ecaborum vendel inctenem dolorem unt vid qui te esequod quos apero que dolorerchil ipiciet volupta vellesti tem hil ipsa volorrovit que vid maxima voluptis quid ut aut odicid mo occumqui conseque nis iur? Sae quossun discimincia sa solor mod ea dusae pelit, tem untur?

Bit erspero vitemodi consed qui dolorerum in perunt.

Aperepero conessincia que es nis ipsumquatem nos dolorerspel int mosa venientiat assumquo occat enim facea nimaiorempos anda con natet et aut quos aut officium, quam

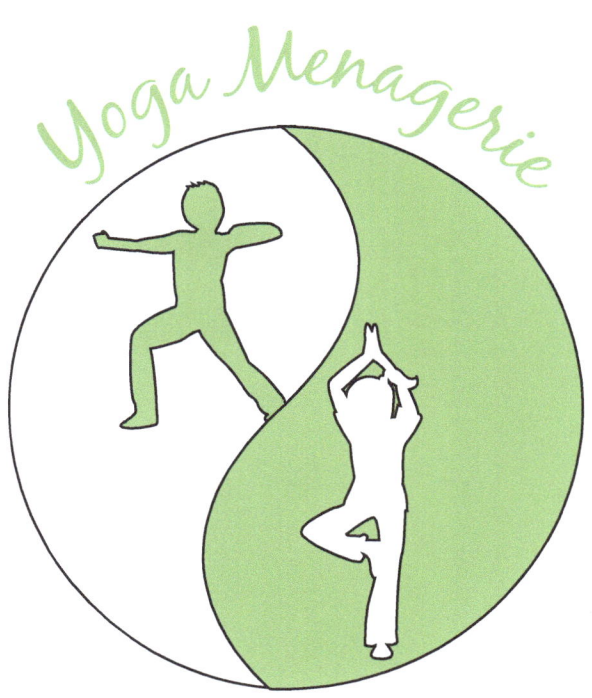